you.

Apostle Dobson

HOW I DEFEATED
CANCER

Ena Dobson

authorHOUSE®

AuthorHouse™
1663 Liberty Drive
Bloomington, IN 47403
www.authorhouse.com
Phone: 1-800-839-8640

First published by AuthorHouse 05/25/2011

ISBN: 978-1-4567-4513-4 (e)
ISBN: 978-1-4567-4514-1 (sc)

Library of Congress Control Number: 2011903882

Printed in the United States of America

Any people depicted in stock imagery provided by Thinkstock are models,
and such images are being used for illustrative purposes only.
Certain stock imagery © *Thinkstock.*

This book is printed on acid-free paper.

Because of the dynamic nature of the Internet, any web addresses or
links contained in this book may have changed since publication and
may no longer be valid. The views expressed in this work are solely those
of the author and do not necessarily reflect the views of the publisher,
and the publisher hereby disclaims any responsibility for them.

This book is dedicated to my Family

My Father, Sidney Harris and my mother, Eulalee Harris, both of whom are still alive . . . I thank God for them. To my husband, Lloyd, who always encourages me and tell me that you can do anything that you put your heart into. Also, to my four children, Dalton: Karen, Nadia, and Veneshia. To my three grandchildren: Jalen, Judane, Je'niya, all of whom loves me and lets me know that life can be anything that I desire.

ACKNOWLEDGMENTS

I first want to acknowledge God Who transformed my life into who I am today. For it is His will that I am alive today and it is Him Who gets all the glory. To my husband, Lloyd, who has been my encourager and to Estella here has been with me from start to finish and she is always speaking spiritually and positively into my life. She is always there when I am encountering hard times and for this I am forever grateful.

To Pastor Eurica Stewart, my good friend and to Ophelia Dawn my spiritual daughters. To Sister Chan, my friend who allowed me to spend quiet time in her home to finish the project of writing this book. I want to tell you Sister Chan that many blessings are awaiting you.

And I will always be grateful to everyone who has helped me in the time of need. May God bless all of you.

Biography of Apostle Dr. Ena Dobson

Dr. Ena Dobson is a wife, a mother of four, as well as a grandmother of three. She is a woman of God and loves God with a passion. She is Holy Spirit filled and she uses her talents in the Lord to help those who are struggling to move forward in their journey with the Lord.

She has been a born again believer for over thirty years and has been in the capacity of a pastor for over ten years. She is a graduate of Canada Christian Bible College and she holds a Bachelor's Degree in Counseling. She also holds a degree in General Practice Psychotherapist. She obtained her Master's Degree in Religious Education and Counseling and was ordained as Clergy with a Certification of Pastoral Counseling in Ontario, Canada.

She has been connected with many ministries in the United States which includes Deeper Life Ministries in Queens, New York under the leadership of Pastor Charles Saddafal. World Harvest Church under the leadership of Pastor Ron Parsley. Tearing Down Walls International Ministries under the leadership of Pastors Larry and Patricia Jackson. Her spiritual mentors Others Pastor Eurica Stewart, Pastor Juliet Wallace, and Rev John Cecil Taylor of Ontario, Canada.

Dr. Dobson recently relocated to the United Stated where

she continues to minister and is launching her counselor's carrier. She has ministered on the Mike Weir Show on WCNO 89.9 on Saturday Night Live. She is a blessing to everyone that she comes in contact with.

At a young age, Ena had an encounter with God that changed her life and she has never forgotten it. According to St. Mark 16: 15 -18, she has traveled to different countries to preach to the sick and they were healed and many were delivered from demonic oppression. God has used Dr. Dobson tremendously and she has touched many lives.

However, in June 2005, she was diagnosed with colon cancer and needless to say, this changed her life dramatically. While in this crucible, she developed tremendous faith in God and that faith manifested and she was healed from cancer and her life was restored.

She is fully persuaded of God's Word and she is dedicated to His purpose for her. She is truly a woman of God. This is her first book and her testimony has helped to build faith and restoration in others. Apostle Dr. Ena Dobson is a dynamic woman of prayer.

Contents

Introduction

*H*ave you ever had a dream and wondered if it would come true? Or have you prayed to God to bring that dream to pass? But then it would sometimes cross your mind that it was just a dream. But dreams are true, but you must wait on the manifestation.

A dream must be something that you should leave for someone else. Never interfere with a dreamer. A dreamer is a romantic. Webster says that a dreamer is an unpractical person. The word of God tells us that we are people.

This reminds me of the story of Joseph and his brothers and how they hated him because he was a dreamer of things to come. Genesis 37: 3-5 says: "***Now Israel loved Joseph more than all his children, because he was the son of his old age: and he made him a coat of many colours. And when his brethren saw that their father loved him more than all his brethren, they hated him, and could not speak peaceably unto him.***

And Joseph dreamed a dream, and he told it his brethren: and they hated him yet the more."

There are times you cannot reveal what you know or what God is saying to you because people will discourage you and even hate you for what they can't have. Everyone at one time or another comes to that conclusion . . . that your dream will come true!

One morning at 3:00 am while I was in bed, I had a visitation from the Lord. He appeared to me and told me to go to the entire world and lay hands on the sick and they shall be delivered in my name (Matthew 16: 18-19).

I got up out of bed and sit down for a few minutes and had to catch my breath for a few minutes because something strange was happening to me and my right hand felt as though it had fire on it. I knew this was not an ordinary experience.

Oftentimes people think I am strange, but they do not understand what is going on in my mind nor do they seek to find out.

It is here that I wrote the vision down just as it stated in Habakkuk 2: 1-3: *"I will stand upon my watch, and set me upon the tower, and will watch to see what he will say unto me, and what I shall answer when I am reproved.*

And the Lord answered me, and said, write the vision, and make it plain upon tables, that he may run that readeth it.

For the vision is yet for an appointed time, but at the end it shall speak, and not lie: though it tarry, wait for it; because it will surely come, it will not tarry."

Chapter One

My Life Begins

From the age of five until I was sixteen, I lived with my grandfather. It seems to me that it was from one extreme to another. My grandfather did not have much; however, he could afford a wife. He was married, but his wife disliked me. She was abusive and oftentimes slapped me for no apparent reason. She thought I knew what she was doing.

I did not realize that I was gifted by God. But oftentimes I would see thing before they happened, and I would tell her. Her response to me was "where do you get these things?"

Now my grandfather was a very hard worker and he would get up early in the morning and go far away to the fields while his wife would take care of their grocery store that they had built from scratch. I watched how she did things and how she dealt with the customers. When the customer would come into the shop, I would help them and do things the exact way she would did them; and she in turn, would tell me how smart I was.

Now, my grandfather loved me dearly, and I could really relate to him. He really understood me, but his wife did not understand me. She was very jealous of our relationship and by slapping me she thought she would make me stay away from my grandfather or that she could at least keep me from getting close to him. But the more she slapped me the closer I drew to him.

As time passed, his business grew larger with livestock and I even got a pet. I named my pet Sheila, she was brown cow and she got to know me well. Because of the business, my uncle which was one of my grandfather's son's came to live with us and that changed everything. No one knew what happened when I was by myself most of the times. My grandmother lived close by and oftentimes I would run to her to spare myself of the beatings. But somehow I came to think that they were my fault.

When I reached nine years of age, my uncle began to make sexual advances towards me. He should have been protecting me, but instead he was molesting me and it left many scars. As I grew older, (most of my life), I believed that being molested was my fault too and I also believed that no one really loved me.

Now the problem was that I could not tell anyone of this matter, because no one would believe me anyway. And on top of all that I was going through, I was being punished physically with the beatings. So I kept being molested a secret.

There were times that I was so angry with all the things that were going on with me as a little girl and this continued until I was a teenager. I never had the opportunity to tell anyone about my situation because my family and friends were in their own little world.

However, all things worked together for my good as the word of God declares. Because of what I have gone through I am able to help others and counsel those who have gone through or are going through the same thing that I went through. There are many times and many places that I have ministered and shared my testimony and people were delivered and set free. John 8: 36 says "***If the Son therefore shall make you free, ye shall be free indeed.***" I would often wonder why all these things were happening to me and I wondered if it was because I was a bad person. Oh, so many questions and no answers that is 'until the Lord showed up.' And as we know, God is never late . . . but He is always on time. He is an on-time God.

On day while I was washing dishes by the river, singing one of the songs I had learned while in Sunday School, I felt this awesome presence and when I turned I saw an angelic being standing over me. I kept this experience a secret because I was afraid no one would believe me. Now in my later years, I realize that, that was bad case of fear. In order for one to understand what others are going through or have been through you usually have had to travel the same route, or have gone through the same trial -- then and only then can you sincerely understand.

Things are not as they are today and many of our dreams die because of lack of knowledge when you don't express yourself. As a little girl being the age of thirteen, I did not want to tell my elders, because I thought that they would just look at me and think that I was losing my mind [and I was probably right]. In my childhood days, like with other children, the pain was almost unbearable.

I used to think that no one cared for me, not even my parents. You see, I did not have nurturing parents. It was only my grandfather that showed love and expressed love for me. And I had the opportunity to know and to understand my grandfather before he passed away. God bless his soul. One of the most important things he instilled in me was the importance of love.

My grandfather was a small frame of a man, approximately 5' 3" tall and from an Indian background. His mother came from India and his father was from the island of Jamaica. When I was a little girl, I never heard a harsh word from him. He never spoke a harsh word to me. He was very loving, sweet, and compassionate. Many would say that I was his favorite child. I truly thank God for his love and care towards me. And he was my mentor at that time in my life.

However, negative thoughts were still in my mind about being unloved. My parents took me back home at the age of sixteen to live with my siblings and we could not get along. We were always fighting and I was quiet and couldn't explain myself; so crying was my answer. Now as I look back and I can see the hand of the Lord upon my life and that I was in this world for a purpose. If the Son therefore shall make you free, ye shall be free indeed.

Now at the age of nineteen there was another incident that happened to me. My mother sent me to see a friend in another place and when I arrived at this place here friend was not there and so I turned to go back home. I had to get on the bus and while waiting on the bus and little boy came up and asked me if I was OK. I cannot remember if I answered him or not, but I do remember lying in someone's house for three hours. When I woke up there were three ladies standing over me. One was dressed in red, the other in royal blue, and the third one in white. They were praying for me and the one in white told me that "we had to pray you back to life."

God spoke to me that day and told me that the three ladies that I saw standing over me praying for me were angels. Never had I seen these ladies before, and after they finished praying for me, they disappeared. That was an experience that never left my mind. The visitation was intense. Now there was one experience after another and fear begin to set in and it drove me. I would keep everything as a secret. The EMENY knew that his time was short in my life so he tried everything in the book to keep me from fulfilling my purpose on earth.

Satan can only form weapons against you, but God always have a better plan for your life.

Chapter Two

The Deception

$\mathcal{I}$ was in a relationship with a man that said he loved me and I was so happy to know that I was getting married. But when you are young and stupid all you see is love [or what you perceive as love]. My grandfather used to say that love is blind. But what I discovered is that love is not blind because God is love (1 John 4:8), because whoever comes into your life will either make you or break you.

When someone tells you that they love you, take time to pray, take time to be watchful and let the relationship grow before marriage. This person said that he really love me, and he even went to my dad and asked for my hand in marriage which was heart breaking because he migrated to the United States and forget what was necessary. It wasn't the plan of God for my life and that didn't last.

At twenty-two I already had a child with no husband, but three months after the birth of my son and not knowing what to do; I did not realize that God was working things out in my life. It was then that I took my son to a Pentecostal

Church and dedicated him to the Lord. God is so good to me. I did not understand my purpose, yet, God was working everything out for my good. I had the opportunity to travel to Canada and this would help my son in the future and I decided that I would not let this opportunity pass me by.

My parents took my son when he was nine months old and this time I trusted my parents to look after him. I didn't know what life had to offer, but I would try to put on a good face even when I was hurting inside.

No matter what others would say to me or what they offered me I would never drink or smoke no matter how they tried to pressure me into it . . . it just was not my style. But on the other hand I was very promiscuous.

It is recorded in statistics that when a person is molested or raped many times they have a tendency of getting into an area of their life that they themselves don't even like. I hated the lifestyle but yet I did not know how to leave it. And even though life seems hard at time, falling into self pity will not help you. Life at time is full of surprises and "all bad things must come to an end." The word of God tells you in Jeremiah 29:11 "***For I know the thoughts that I think toward you, saith the Lord, thoughts of peace, and not of evil, to give you an expected end.***" But I was ignorant of this promise given to me by God and that is what Satan had over me. I did not know that God had a better plan for my life. God has a plan for every individual on this earth, and His plan is for you to know and understand your purpose.

At this time, I got married to a friend that I had known since high school. I married because I thought that it would ease the pain. However, it only made things worse. Running from God is not a nice thing because while you are running, you are missing out on the beautiful things God has for you. He wants you to have the best in life. How it ends depends on how it begins. And you have to eventually come to that decision one way or another.

Through this time of running, I had many visitations from the Lord that I have not forgotten even to this day. When you run away from God, He will catch up with you in His time and even more so if He calls you to do His will. You will find out that your will must surrender to His will and His way and not your way of thinking or reasoning.

The Lord wants to help someone who will desire to read and persevere in their lives. There were times when I tried to take my life by swallowing pills to ease the pain. I tried it again and again, but it did not work.

The day came when I finally yielded to the Lord and during this time I was out under the power of God for three and a half hours. During this time I had many visions. I saw a shepherd with a staff in His hand and He was feeding the sheep and the shepherd told me to go and feed My sheep. Every since I came out of that atmosphere my life has not been the same, even to this day.

I realize that all that time God was drawing me to the kingdom for such a time as this. You see, I was living according to the flesh. My way of thinking opposed to God's word. When you choose to live this way, you open the door for Satan to draw you away from the will of God for your life. To prevent this, you must allow the word of Good to be the final authority in your life and thus, the word of God will cast down Satan's suggestions.

Satan made a suggestion to Eve in the Garden of Eden to tempt her to doubt what God had already said (Genesis

3: 1-5). Satan's will is to weaken your defenses by making suggestions to you. When negative thoughts come, immediately cast them down with the word of God. Don't give the enemy any place in your mind; don't even consider his suggestions. He wants you to listen to his words so that your thinking and emotions will be affected so that you will make decisions outside of the will of God for your life.

Eve listened to Satan's words and gave in to his suggestion to eat fruit of the tree of knowledge of good and evil (Gen. 3:6). As a result of Adam's and Eve disobedience, the blessing departed and a curse was invited onto the earth.

You were not created to operate outside of God's word. His word outlines the purpose for everything in life. And when you don't allow the Bible to be your guideline for living, you will open Satan's lies regarding life and how you should operate. It is a choice you have to make for yourself; no one can do that for you. And it is called self-control. People that can't control themselves will try to control others. If I can get a grip on my thinking and if my thinking is right with God then my emotions will be right, thus, I will line up with the word of God and have peace on the inside. Thus, you will be walking in the will of God, and you know that every thought, movement, and every word of Christ is targeted for a divine purpose. Walking after the flesh will destroy your life.

The "flesh" is a way of thinking that opposes God's word. To be spiritual is to have life and peace, which brings a rest that will be in your spirit. To walk according to the word of God will bring you great success and blessings will also follow you. No one will be able to take from you, and the love of God will be manifested in your life as you grow in faith. Without faith it was impossible to please God, for the word says that I was to believe, and then I would receive.

Most of the time I spent flipping through the Bible seeking for what God's word says about my life, and that's where I was searching to get answers. Jeremiah 1:10 says: "***See, I have this day set thee over the nations and over the kingdoms, to root out, and to pull down, and to destroy, and to throw down, to build, and to plant.***"

I realize that from a young age the Lord was calling me. I would hear my name and totally ignore it. At thirteen years of age an angel of the Lord appeared to me while I was washing dishes at the river. The presence of the Lord came upon me, but I was afraid to go into the church or tell anyone.

You can only run for so long but you can't hide. Many are called but few are chosen. I know that some things don't come easy. Many times people would look at me as if they had seen a ghost. People would pretend that they loved me for a moment then after a while they started to ignore me. There are times that I cried myself to sleep.

For years a spirit of rejection hovered over me and would not leave me until I came into the knowledge of spiritual things. The truth of the matter is rejection is very painful and if you are not delivered from that spirit you can be very bitter, hateful and resentful and it will finally destroy you.

Out of that painful lifestyle there can come a greater ministry. Your pain and agony will help someone else receive deliverance. Some times what we go through is a benefit to other for what they are going through or what they will be going through. It takes a lot of sacrifices that many are not willing to make. It is to know Me, Jesus said in the power of His resurrection and in the fellowship of suffering.

You can't say you love Jesus and go through life without partaking in His suffering. We are at the end-times and Jesus coming is very soon and many of our children don't even know Jesus Christ as their personal Savior.

As a single mother with four children and no husband, it wasn't easy. But as I look back now, I realize that the Lord was with me all along. I had no job because I hurt my back and couldn't work. I had to get on welfare with my children and once a week went to the food bank so that my children would not go hungry. I did not let my circumstances stop me. I was determined to follow my divine destiny. People put me down and said many negative things about me, but yet I pressed my way through.

My first step was going back to school which I did and graduated with a degree in Fashion Design. I proved everyone wrong that was talking about me and putting me down. I will not tell you that it was easy. My children told me "Mom, you can do it." My children encouraged me and they saw what others could not see in me. I noticed that many of my friends were not happy for me, as a matter of fact; they were jealous . . . but to God be the glory. It is God Who brought me through. Who can stop you when God is ordering your step? Whom God blesses let no man curse.

Chapter Three

My Children's Love

My oldest son is thirty-seven years old and God has called him to preach the gospel. I can remember when he was nine years old and he preached his first sermon. On that night, many lives were changed and many times he would go to places with me to pray for people. He was never afraid of demons. It would be his pleasure to help me pray. I see the call of God on his life and that helped me press forward because I was realizing that my whole life depends on Jesus. Being a single parent is easy, but my son was like a husband, he was constantly worrying about my well being.

He and I had a good relationship and he never hid anything from me. He would watch my life and he asked questions all the time. When he was eleven years of age, he was just getting into high school. I had got laid off of job and at this time Christmas was right around the corner. My son went to school and saw to it that his mother and sisters would have gifts for Christmas.

Unfortunately, my son walked away from the Lord. As a

matter of fact, he ran away from God. But he may run, but he cannot hide. Because God made me a promise and he would preach the gospel. I am constantly praying and believing, because I am reminded of the promises that God has made in His word. The passion that my son once had is going to be restored again; more than he had the first time. I don't care what the devil does; my son will preach the gospel.

God gave me an idea of adopting other children and to pray for them while others pray for my children. The Bible teaches us to pray one for another. I am grateful for the opportunity God has given me as I travel and minister across this world and for sure, God is working on my behalf.

My oldest daughter is thirty-five years old. When I was pregnant with her, her father didn't want anything to do with the pregnancy. As a matter of fact he told me that I should have an abortion. Honestly, I thought about it because life was hard with me being in another country. I had no family, hardly any friends. I didn't know the Lord and my job was not what I wanted. Looking back now, I can see the love of God with me at all times. My daughter was born and at six weeks old I had to board her out with a family so that I could go back to work. I thought that was the best thing to do, but my heart was hurting because I wanted to see my daughter make her first steps which I am sure that every mother desires that.

I did not know that my daughter's spine had a curvature in her lower back which caused a lot of problems. But through it all, the Lord has been good to us and we learned how to cope with the situation. She also had a speech impediment which the Lord brought her through after she went through extensive therapy. And again, I can see the hand of the Lord at work in my family.

She was able to finish high school believing God for greater things to happen in her life. I watched her love the Lord and develop a powerful prayer life. She did not let what was going on around her stop her. Sometimes I thought it was my fault why my daughter suffered this infirmity.

One day a man of God ministered to us and told me "it's not your fault what your daughter is going through; God is going to fix all of that." Luke 13:16 says that Jesus loosed the women whom Satan had bound for eighteen years. I believe that God has a set time for my daughter to complete what He has started.

My Third Child

My child, Pat, was a little runner and still is. The reason why I make that statement is that from my pregnancy [from start to finish], it was like she was playing football in my womb and it seemed to be non-stop. I started bleeding through my nostrils and that caused me to stop working at an early time in the pregnancy.

With proper rest, she was born on the very date that the doctor gave. The moment I went into labor she was born while I was going to the hospital. Yes, she was coming out in the automobile and the police had to escort us to the hospital. This child always loved excitement. Even to this day, when she steps into a room, it lights up with her presence.

At an early age, we were in church where the Holy Spirit was moving. And as we were praising God she was speaking in tongues and she was only five years old. God gave her a voice to sing for His glory. My sister is a Christian today because of this child. Again, the hand of the Lord was at work in my children's lives.

Six Years Later

We were out doing some summer shopping. And as I went into the children's store, the Lord spoke to me that I will need this particular set of clothing. My response was "I don't need these clothes." Little did I know that I was pregnant with a child again after six years.

One day while I was praying, God spoke to me and told me that "this child that you are carrying will be different from all the children you have had." "What was the difference?" I asked as I was on my knees. Well, I was constantly in warfare with her. One morning at 4:00 am I was awaken by an angelic being touching my stomach and she started moving rapidly in me.

As time approach for delivery, my water broke for a week, but yet the baby would not come. I was two days past due, and my mother who was living with me, begin to pray for the baby to arrive. The baby was born, but when she came her skin looked like an old lady's skin. She was all wrinkled up, yet again; I saw the hand of the Lord at work for His divine purpose in our lives.

At an early age, she was baptized and filled with the Holy Spirit. At the age of nine, she could play the keyboard by just listening to a song.

I give the Lord praise for His goodness. The hand of the Lord is on all my children. Psalm 127: 3-5 says "***Lo, children are an heritage of the Lord: and the fruit of the womb is his reward.***

As arrows are in the hand of a mighty man; so are children of the youth.

Happy is the man that hath his quiver full of them: they shall not be ashamed, but they shall speak with the enemies in the gate."

There is nothing more beautiful that you serving the Lord in gladness. I surrendered my life to God over thirty years ago, to walk in the covenant blessing with the Father. He has placed His Spirit within us to give us power and authority over the power of the air. Luke 10:19 says: "**<u>Behold, I give unto you power to tread on serpents and scorpions, and over all the power of the enemy: and nothing shall by any means hurt you.</u>**" This means you have "dunamis" power for working miracles. God gave us power to work with. He has given you tools. You are not alone.

My husband and my friend Marie encourages me to go to Bible School. She was going to the same Bible School that blessed me very much, because this was a dream come true. As we studied, she reminded me that I can do all things through Christ who strengthened me. Many times in class I would feel the presence of God in class. I would be inspired with His grace which brought forth love and passion for God's purpose on earth.

I was ordained as a Pastor in 1999. I was a graduate at Canada Christian Bible College where I received my Bachelor Degree in Counseling. My husband's obedience to God later led me to the World Harvest Church, where I received godly teaching and instruction under the guidance of Pastor Rod Parsley, one of my spiritual mentors.

In 1985 my friend and I went to New York to visit a ministry of deliverance, and it was there that I saw a lot of people set free by the power of God. My life was a challenge because part of my calling was to set captives free.

I was training for ten years in Deeper Life Ministry by Dr. Charles Saddafel and he was one of my mentors. He trained us well and whoever trained under this man of God came out with tremendous testimonies.

The people would come out for deliverance and went everywhere Jesus went, and He was doing good healing for all those who were oppressed with devils for God was with Him. 2 Corinthians 7:1 says: "*Having therefore these promises, dearly beloved, let us cleanse ourselves from all filthiness of the flesh and spirit, perfecting holiness in the fear of God.*" 2 Timothy 2:21 says: "*If a man therefore purge himself from these, he shall be a vessel unto honour, sanctified, and meet for the master's use, and prepared unto every good work.*"

It's always a privilege looking for more learning because it's never too much. There is always room for more when you are hungry for the things of God. Looking forward to graduating from Bible School was one of the most exciting times of my life. I studied hard and I felt like a little girl again and all my dreams were coming to past.

I always dreamed dreams. Many of those dreams were manifesting. I always would feel like Joseph the dreamer, when he would tell his brothers and they hated him and sold him into slavery. Yet in all this, God used that evil action of humans to work out His will in Joseph's life. Those who fear

God and acknowledge Him in their ways have the promise that God will direct all their steps (Proverbs 3: 5-7).

I was praising God all the way through because it was only God that helped me through those long nights of studying when my life was like a journey.

There are times in a person's life when you think all is well and you are untouchable, but that's when everything goes downhill. I felt strong because that was my nature. I always believed if I would go after something and worked hard at it, it would come to pass.

Prayer was my lifeline. A lady, who was going to the same Bible School that I went to, came to me and made this statement: "Did you hear that everything starts in the colon?" My reply was: "I don't know about that," but I wondered what she was referring to and knowing that I was really hearing the word 'cancer.'

Now when I first got that news, the word that came to mind is death and it is right here that you have to overcome the fear and defeat. Death wasn't an option, but it was a life for me. I prayed and interceded for God to heal me. I felt like Daniel when he prayed. From the first day his prayer was answered, but the prince of the kingdom of Persia who is the devil, Satan himself, held back the answer from coming forth.

I had prayed for many people that God had healed and now asked the question "Why not me?" The answer came "Why not you" it wasn't easy, so I submitted to God's will that He can have His way in me. Sometimes you must be careful of what you pray for because it might not go the way you expect it to. God has to get His glory out of your life.

This atmosphere allowed me to develop a passion for the things of God in more depth in my spiritual life. People everywhere was praying for me. I truly thank God for the people that He had placed in my life. I had to go through the surgery and the doctor told me that he had removed sixteen lymph nodes and four were cancerous. The doctor told us that I was in the third stage.

Many times I would think to myself maybe it was something I had done or desired because I did not know it was just a process of getting me closer to God.

After this surgery I stayed in the hospital for six day. In the hospital I had the opportunity to minister to this lady and led her to the Lord. She told me I was her angel sent from the Lord and I know the Lord was pleased because His will was accomplished. Jesus for this same purpose destroyed the work of the devil. John 3:8 says: "*He that committeth sin is of the devil; for the devil sinneth from the beginning. For this purpose the Son of God was manifested, that he might destroy the works of the devil.*" Just as Jesus came for sinners, it should be the same for our souls. "*And whithersoever he entered, into villages, or cities, or country, they laid the sick in the streets, and besought him that they might touch if it were but the border of his garment: and as many as touched him were made whole*" (Mark 6:56).

"*Come unto me, all ye that labour and are heavy laden, and I will give you rest*" (Matt. 11:28). When you are burden down you carry a heavy load worrying about responsibility of difficult duties with the burden of parenthood. Many families are walking in this type of burden. I have noticed this everywhere I go. It takes the anointing of God's power to break this type of power in the earth. The ship's capacity is the maximum weight of cargo that the ship can carry. Without Jesus, you will be like a ship without a captain. The captain needs Jesus direction all the way, especially when there are any disturbances. If not the ship will sink and everyone who lives on that ship will die. Life and death is in the power of the tongue, speak life.

Chapter Four

My Going Home

After those days spent in the hospital, I discharged thinking that was freedom until I got home, and that's where the trouble really began in my life. My first day home from the hospital was not what I expected, because the infection set in and I got nervous. My husband and children were also afraid about the infection because it begins to pour out of the wound that I had in my belly. It wasn't a nice sight. I had to be rushed back to the hospital for a second time. Even with all his happening, I was holding to the word which was in my heart *"I shall not die, but live, and declare the works of the Lord"* (Ps. 118:17).

I was confident in God and that He was going to see me through. I know that Jehovah Rapha is my healer and as I realized this, nothing else mattered. God was going to bring my deliverance. My weakest days were my strongest and the word of God was my meat. I would listen to the word of God everyday and repeat and confess the healing Scriptures over my body and continue to say my confession and to believe Him to bring me out of this situation.

After six weeks, I started to see the progress of God setting me free. The Word of God says in John 8:36 " *If the Son therefore shall make you free, ye shall be free indeed.*" Nothing is more foundational to your freedom from Satan's bondage than understanding and affirming what God has done for you in Christ and who you are as His child. Your attitude, action, response and reactions of life circumstances are greatly affect by you and affirming what God has done for you in Christ, and who you are as His child and your beliefs about yourself as directed in Ephesians 5:19.

If you see yourself as helpless victims of Satan and his schemes, you will live like a victim and you will be in bondage to his lies. Satan is the father of lies and his desire is to wreck you. And if you give in to his lies then you will be defeated.

I had made up my mind to press in for victory. It wasn't easy because first and foremost you have to win the battle in your mind which is the battle ground. Nothing really comes easy. You have to tell yourself that you are a winner at all times.

My Healing Started

I started reading prophecy Scriptures over my life that Jesus said in His word. Every day I learned how to declare by what comes out of my mouth (positive or negative) faith or unbelief " And I will give unto thee the keys of the kingdom of heaven: and whatsoever thou shalt bind on earth shall be bound in heaven: and whatsoever thou shalt loose on earth shall be loosed in heaven" (Matthew 16:19). "*Thou shalt also decree a thing, and it shall be established unto thee*" (Job 2:28). Isaiah 53:4 says: "*Surely he hath borne our griefs, and carried our sorrows: yet we did esteem him stricken, smitten of God, and afflicted.*" Proverbs 3:24 says: "*When thou liest down, thou shalt not be afraid: yea, thou shalt lie down, and thy sleep shall be sweet.*"

"*There remaineth therefore a rest to the people of God. For he that is entered into his rest, he also hath ceased from his own works, as God did from his. Let us labour therefore to enter into that rest, lest any man fall after the same example of unbelief*" (Heb. 4: 9-11).

Many times I am encouraged that I am a fighter, and until I started walking in that belief nothing would happen. And I press toward the high calling of God in Christ Jesus. There was a time when I felt as if death was at my door because of all the medication I had to take. One of the main Scriptures that would help me was Psalm 23: 1-6: "*The Lord is my shepherd; I shall not want.*

He maketh me to lie down in green pastures: he leadeth me beside the still waters.

He restoreth my soul: he leadeth me in the paths of righteousness for his name's sake.

Yea, though I walk through the valley of the shadow of death, I will fear no evil: for thou art with me; thy rod and thy staff they comfort me.

Thou preparest a table before me in the presence of mine enemies: thou anointest my head with oil; my cup runneth over.

Surely goodness and mercy shall follow me all the days

of my life: and I will dwell in the house of the Lord for ever."

All of these healing Scriptures were so close to my heart and I would read them and study them every day until the word became a part of me. Many times I had to go for medication and I would sleep for days and could do nothing. And that bothered me because I knew that I was not a lazy person. This would just eat away at me, but my friends told me that I was going to be OK.

As I said before, my sister, Estella was a big part of my life. She would call me every day. Sometimes three times a day to see if I was ok even though she was not living in the same state that I lived in [I was constantly on her mind]. She would prophecy over me and encourage me; and for that I am grateful. My friend and pastor, Pastor Stewart came to see me in the hospital while had a needle in my vein in my right arm. She went home and told the Lord that she needed an answer to her prayer unto Him. She said Lord, please do not take her, she is like the sister that I never had. **"... Ask me of things to come concerning my sons, and concerning the work of my hands command ye me"** (Isaiah 45:11). "**The Lord is my strength and my shield; my heart trusted in him, and I am helped**" (Psalms 28:7).

It is God Who is giving you help. Matthew 7:8 says: "**for every one that asketh receiveth; and he that seeketh findeth; and to him that knocketh it shall be opened**." "**But the Lord is faithful, who shall stablish you, and keep you from evil**" (2 Thess. 3:3). "**The fear of the Lord tendeth to life: and he that hath it shall abide satisfied; he shall not be visited with evil**" (Proverbs 19:23). While I was confessing those words God was doing His part in me. Every day, I had a port that was put over my right breast that has left me with a scar until this day. From this experience I developed a deep passion in my spiritual walk with the Lord.

Nothing can every change my mind from believing that God is real. Many ask me the questions "how do you do it?" My answer is it took everything that is within me and more. I pressed through and continued confessing the word and praising God for His goodness towards me. The desire became intensity for God like never before.

I had the desire of drinking green juice and so I had this juicer that you can juice the things and drink. Doing so wasn't a problem because my stomach would digest it. So by doing this, my white cell counts (neutrophilis) and my red cell count (hemoglobin) was reproducing every time. I would receive a chemo session and the cells would be normal. It worked, and I would encourage others that have the same condition to do as I did and they would get the same results.

We were told that your intake of food should be more protein which was inclusive of calories, increase of fluids, servings of fruit and vegetables, high fiber. This food would improve your blood count. And that along with getting rest and exercise would improve your health. I was learning how to even fast through this. These were my options for survival. If I was to live a normal life, I would eat a little of everything.

I was told that side effects will come because of the chemo. And, of course, it did. At times, I was weak, tired, dizzy, nauseated, vomiting, teeth bleeding, hair loss, change of complexion, and my mouth would be so sore that at times nothing I would eat would even have taste. At times I would feel so bad that I know only God Himself understands what an individual goes through in these times.

Because of the courses that I had taken, I was not taking counseling and I was able to cope with many of the problems that faced me. One of the ways I was dealing with this traumatic experience seeking help from Christ Jesus . . . in the sense of full surrender to Christ. I recognized that I could not face this part of my life on my own. My husband played a big part and also some of my close friends who would not give up on me and that encouraged me even when I felt as if I was going crazy. My husband would say to me "get your focus on God and know that He is with you." And again, for this reason, I would say to myself: 'let the fire of God burn within you.' These things would go through my mind. But I would have a burning desire to please God. It is not matter what I would see, the Lord would speak to me and say "I am with you."

I asked myself "what is desire?" It is a natural longing that is excited by the enjoyment or the thought of any good that implies you to action or efforts in its continuance or possession; an eager wish to obtain or enjoy.

Unspeakable desire is to see, know and express a wish or request a petition. My mother said and yield and consent to the desire. Craving, inclination, eagerness, aspiration, to also long for a wish for earnestly, or to covet. Whatever you desire when you pray, believe that you will have it. Anything which is a desire, an object of longing. Haggai 2:7 says: "***and I will shake all nations, and the desire of all nations shall come: and I will fill this house with glory, saith the Lord of hosts.***" One of my greatest desires is to see God's glory fill the earth in the lives of people. If I could take out my heart and give it, I could only imagine how the Lord feels about His people.

Be Self-Controlled and Alert

One of the most important things that a solider learns in his training is to be alert. He must constantly be watching and on guard for any attack of the enemy. As Christians, we must always be on the alert. We cannot afford to allow the enemy to take us by surprise.

JESUS has commanded that you "WATCH and PRAY that ye enter not into temptation; the spirit indeed is will but the flesh is weak" (Matthew 26:41). Not only are we commanded to WATCH and PRAY, to use prayer as an offensive weapon to prepare us for the battles we face, but God has also called us to watch and prayer for our brothers and sisters through the body of Christ.

The Apostle Paul, after admonishing the Ephesians to put on the armor of God listed various pieces of armor and concluded by saying "*praying always with all prayer and supplication in the Spirit, and watching thereunto with all perseverance and supplication for all saints*" (Ephesians 6:18). We must utilize our weapon of prayer and use it as an OFFENSIVE weapon to be on the alert, to pray without ceasing (1 Thess. 5:17). To persevere in prayer for your fellow soldiers in Canada, United States and other nations on the earth.

You must not take this responsibility lightly. As a soldier praying for your fellow soldier is not an option, it is a requirement. There are other Christians whose lives depend upon prayers, who are risking their jobs, families, their lives for the sake of the Gospel. There are soldiers who have been "wounded" who are tired and are at the point of giving up, that need to be strengthened by your prayers.

There are soldiers whose lives are in danger and nations that are plagued by political turmoil and strife. There are new brothers and sisters who have accepted the Lord and are still behind prison bars. These men and women are living in the midst of the strongholds of the enemy, of fear, hate, and all kinds of perversions. They need the strength of our prayers to uphold them.

I know that God has called me to be a spiritual "watchman." I have been watching because many times the Lord will show me a face of my brothers or sisters. And I realize that the prayer "watchman" sometimes hardly sleeps because you are oftentimes on an assignment praying for somebody. Jesus said in His words "Watch ye therefore, and pray always."

When I was diagnosed with colon cancer, many thought that I would not be alive today. Oftentimes when I see people they look at me strange as if God don't answer prayers. God is merciful, but He will do almost anything to get our attention. Why? Because He loves us. God made a promise to His people Israel that after they experience His judgment they will experience revival of spiritual life and restoration of purpose and blessing.

You want to experience revival! What price have you paid to see such a move? How big is your price? How willing are you to pay that cost? It's not an easy task but one must be willing to pay. Nothing anyone goes through is easy. But in all you go through, you must give thanks for it is the will of God concerning us. My best times in life, is when I am giving thanks. It does something to your spirit man; it causes your spirit to constantly be renewed. We must get back to the basics by renewing our prayer and worship. (Ps. 149: 1-9). God has a plan for you that will affect change not only in your life, but in your neighborhood and in the nations.

The Word foreknown is 'now glorification' which is the noun of glory. It means make glorious, make (common or inferior thing) seem more splendid than it is invested with radiance. Foreknow in the verse is equivalent to (fore love) and is used in the sense of "to set loving upon, to choose to bestow love upon from eternity."

Genesis 18:19 says: "***For I know him, that he will command his children and his household after him, and they shall keep the way of the Lord, to do justice and judgment; that the Lord may bring upon Abraham that which he hath spoken of him***." I know that the way of the Lord is essential in the calling of Abraham. It was God's purpose that he be a spiritual leader at home and teaches children the way of the Lord. One is responsible to train their children in the way of the Lord.

Foreknowledge means that God's purpose for eternity was to love and redeem the human race through Christ. The recipient of God's foreknowledge or fore love is stated in plural and refers to the church. That is, God's fore love is primarily for the body of Christ and individuals only as they identify themselves with this body through abiding faith and union with Christ (1 John 4:19).

Chapter Five

My Growing Up Days

Most of my childhood days were not so pleasant. Wherein most families had their siblings to play with and have fun, life was mostly difficult for me. At the age of five I was sent to live with my grandparents. My grandfather loved me dearly; however, it was still lonely.

I knew that I had sisters, but I did not have the opportunity to be with them, and I that the question of "why?" was stuck in my mind for many years. Now I would spend time with my real parents, but it would only be for short periods of time, then I would be sent back to my grandfather again.

My step grandmother did not love me at all, but she would pretend to love me when my grandfather was around. She would whip me even when there was no need for it. To this day I have scars on my body from the whipping I received from her. And of course, I would cry and I thought that no one cared about me. The pain was almost unbearable, and only God knew what I was going through.

God had a plan for my life. As I grew older, my heart was tender and compassionate toward people; even though many times I would still get hurt from the ones that I loved. I loved my parents very much and many times it would appear that they didn't care and that I was just a mistake. I realize now that the devil put these thoughts in my mind and wanted me to focus on them. I thought that my parents loved my sisters much more than they loved me, and no one could convince me that, that was not so.

Anyone who reads this book, I want you to understand and not take the message out of context, but everything that is written in this book is the information of this book.

It took a while, but I have forgiven my parents. I let resentment and bitterness fester in my heart. I had to let it go, because I could not make good decision because I was looking back into the past all the time. I had to realize that I came into this world to touch the lives of many people.

As a young child I never deserved what I really went through. I was abused by one family who has died now. But as a little girl I felt the abuse, and the bruised marks are still on my body to this day. I was also molested by another member of the family. This was kept secret for many years because no one believed me. It would appear that I was selfish because I did not talk much. I was in mental and emotional pain that no one knew about.

I got an opportunity to spend time with my parents and my siblings. But it wasn't enough when we were together, because there was no peace and we would fight so much and this made me feel like a stranger. At the age of nine years old I was molested and other members of the family tried the same method on me. As a result of this, I would keep to myself and cry.

By the age of thirteen, God visited me at my grandfather's house and that made me afraid, and I would not tell anyone about it. When I was sixteen years of age, my step grandmother had enough of me and she decided to send me back to my parents. I still would not tell anyone of the pain that I was going through, and I would pretend that all was well while my heart was breaking in pieces one incident after another.

I felt so violated and I didn't know who to talk to or who would understand my deepest thoughts. I had actually become suicidal at times and I also could not have a healthy relationship because I would begin to feel violated and on top of everything else, I felt rejected.

Chapter Six

How to Overcome Hurts

Below are the **WRONG WAYS to overcome hurt:**

1. Decide to hurt others. This is the WRONG way to handle hurt. You are not going to get anywhere by hurting someone because you are working in a principle that says: "***give, and it shall be given unto you; good measure, pressed down, and shaken together, and running over, shall men give into your bosom. For with the same measure that ye mete withal it shall be measured to you again***" (Luke 6:38).

2. Harden our hearts: If your heart is hard you cannot hear God because God cannot speak to you if your heart is hardened. You cannot have meaningful relationships and you become a prisoner of your own pain because you have hardened your own heart. (Hebrews 3:8).

3. Pretend we are not really hurt. That's the wrong

way to handle it. Even in a marriage you pretend that you are not hurt, this puts you out of touch with reality and it invites more mistreatment in your life.

4.   Decide not to trust anyone anymore. When you refuse to trust anyone you become paranoid and suspicious of everyone you come in contact with.

5.   Everyone in your life and anyone that can do you good won't be able to do good because you have decided not to trust anyone.

Right Ways to Deal with Hurt and Pain:

1.   Put on the shield of faith: *"above all, taking the shield of faith, wherewith ye shall be able to quench all the fiery darts of the wicked"* (Ephesians 6:16). I know what the shield of faith will do, because we know that without the Word we can't have faith; because faith comes from the Word of God. *"Now faith is the substance of things hoped for, the evidence of things not seen"* (Hebrews 11:1). So the Word of God is equal to faith that you can see and that what the shield of faith is on. When you take the shield of faith and lift it up in your heart faith that you can see and that what the shield of faith is on. When you take the shield of faith and lift it up in your heart you release your burden. You will never be hurt when you have your shield of faith. So when the dart of hurt comes, it will not penetrate your life because you have lifted

your shield of faith and you have the word of
God. You have focus and priority in your life
and in your vault.

The Word of God says more about your life than what
somebody else can say about you. And what they say about
you will not hurt you because the shield of faith is in your
life. When we listen to what other people say about us, we
put our shield down. As soon as we make what they say more
important than what God says, we have lowered our shield
of faith. Then as a result, whatever they told us become our
shield and that is not enough to protect you.

When you suffer from rejection it's not an easy task. No
one knows the pain that I had for years. You would have
to experience that type of situation in order to understand
someone else's pain. Understanding the biblical side of
rejection is a bad spirit that will make you lose. The mind
will keep that kind of behavior as long as you let it. But it
had to be a choice you made.

Life has Certain Principles

1. Our intimacy with God should be the highest
    priority for our lives and it should determine the
    impact of our lives.

2. Obey God and leave all the consequences to
    Him.

3. God's word is an immovable anchor in times
    of storm.

4. The awareness of God's presence energizes us
    for His work.

5. God does not require us to understand His will. Just obey it, even if it seems unreasonable.

6. You reap what you sow, more than you sow and later than you have sown.

7. The dark moments of our life last only as long as is necessary for God to accomplish His purpose in us.

8. Fight all your battles on your knees and win the war every time.

9. Trusting God means looking beyond what we can see to what God sees in you.

10. If necessary, God will move heaven and earth to show us His will.

11. God assumes full responsibility for our needs when we obey Him.

12. Peace with God is the fruit of oneness with God.

13. Listening to God is essential to walking with God.

14. God acts on behalf of those who wait on Him.

15. Brokenness is God's requirement for maximum usefulness.

16. Whatever you acquire outside of God's will eventually turns to nothing. 17. We stand tallest and strongest on our knees.

17. As children of a sovereign God, we are never victims of our circumstances.

18. Anything you hold tightly, you will lose.

19. Disappointments are inevitable, discouragement is a choice.

20. Obedience always bring blessing.

21. To walk in the Spirit is to obey the initial prompting of the Spirit.

22. You can never out give God.

23. To live a Christian life is to allow Jesus to let His life in and through us.

24. God bless us that we might bless others.

25. Adversity is a bridge to a deeper relationship with God.

26. Prayer is life's greatest time saver.

27. No Christian has ever been called to "do it alone" in his or her walk of faith.

28. We learn more in our valley experiences than on our mountain tops.

29. An eager anticipation of the Lord's return keeps us living productively.

A friend told me one day that Enoch walked with God, and that was how I would have to walk. I wondered what she was talking about. Then as I studied the Word of God and as time went by, others told me the same thing. I learned from a dear friend of mine and she prayed from me so much and the Lord spoke to her one day that I am the female side of Enoch. That put a fear in me so much the more. No one at times understands me; some even make fun of me; and other agrees with me; yet others are not happy with me . . . but life goes on. "And Enoch walked with God: and he was not; for God took him" (Gen. 5:24).

Enoch was the father of the long lived Methuselah and the great grandfather of Noah. It is said that he walked with God after the birth of Methuselah, three hundred years. It was a long time for a man to support a holy life and communion with God without any relapse worthy of notice.

It is difficult for Christians now to do this for a single day. How remarkable then that he have done it for the long space of three hundred years.

Such approval did his extraordinary piety gain him, that when the time came for him to leave the world, God transformed him, as He afterwards did Elijah and suffered him not to taste the bitterness of death. Perhaps to show mankind what he would have done for them had he never sinned.

Some shine in all brilliancy of marital achievements, and are renowned for the conquest of kingdoms. Others have gathered laurels in the path of science and illumined the world with flashes of their genius. Others by their counsels have swayed the fate of empires, and the deeds of these have been loudly sounded by the trumpet of fame. But more is said in praise of this man of God in a few short words of our text, than is said of them all. A greater character is given him in four words, than is ascribed to the most renowned warriors and statement by the whole voice of history and poetry. There is something very expressive in the phrase, "I walked with God."

The Christian life is frequently called a walk, and believers are exhorted to walk circumspectly, not as fools but as wise. It is called walking before God; I remember now how I have walked before thee in truth." The figure of walking before God was drawn perhaps from the position of those who worshipped in the tabernacle and temple. The Shekinah or visible glory of God sat enthroned on the mercy seat.

The worshippers stood in the outer court directly before the Shekinah, hence the common expression of appearing before God in public worship. To walk before God meant then to lead a life of devotion. But Enoch walked with God. I do not find this character ascribed to any but Enoch and Noah.

I will:

1. Explain what is meant by this figure;

2. Show the consequences of walking with God;

3. State the prominent means by which such a walk can be kept up.

4. Explain accordingly.

It seems to be expensive of something more intimate than the phrase to walk *before* God.

We all know what it is for two friends to walk together, engaged in close and interesting conversation. And this is the figure by which is represented the intercourse of Enoch with his God for three hundred years. The figure is well adapted. The hidden life of the Christian, his retired habit of devotion, his separation from the world, (living, as it were, in the other world while dwelling in this,) his daily, intimate, unseen communion with God, are very fitly represented by two intimate friends walking together, engrossed with each other, unmindful of all the world besides, unseeing and unseen. This general thought comprehends several particulars.

1. When two friends thus walk together their communion is *secret. So is* the communion between the Christian and his God. The world wonders what the Christian finds to employ himself about when alone. They wonder what supports him under trials, and renders his countenance cheerful when they looked for sadness. Let them know then that he draws his comforts from another world; that he lives far away from this, where the changes and trials of the present state do not reach him. As well might they wonder whence Abraham and David derive their present joys, while clouds are darkening the world below.

2. When two friends thus walk together, their *conversation is kind and sweet.* So the man who walks with God pours into his Father's ear all his desires and complaints, and receives his kind and comforting answers in return.

3. When two friends thus walk together their *wills and governing feelings are the same;* for how "can two walk together except they be agreed?" They also keep the same course, and thus are advancing towards the *same object. So* the man who walks with God is conformed to him in

moral character. Benevolence reigns in his heart, and his open arms embrace the universe. Like God, his feelings are in accordance with the holy law. He loves righteousness and hates iniquity. His object too is the same with his. The glory of his Father, the prosperity of Zion, and the happiness of the universe, constitute the one indivisible object of his pursuit. He is delighted with the government of God, and has no controversy with him who shall reign. His will is swallowed up in the divine will. He wishes not to select for himself, but in everything chooses that his heavenly Father should select for him. He is "careful for nothing, but in everything by prayer and supplication, with thanksgiving," makes his "requests known unto God. And the peace of God which passes all understanding, "keeps his heart and mind "through Christ Jesus."There are two other things implied in walking with God which are not exactly suggested by the figure.

1. The man who walks with God walks *humbly.* God will not walk with him else; for "the proud he knoweth afar off." The whole of man's duty is summed up in doing justly, in loving mercy, and in walking "humbly" with his God. The Christian, with all his intimacy with his Maker, does not approach him with familiar boldness, but is the more abased the more ho sees of him. "I have heard of thee," said Job, "by the hearing of the ear, but now my eye seeth thee; wherefore I abhor myself and repent in dust and ashes."

2. The man who walks with God exercises a living

faith. This, according to the apostle, was the main spring of all those graces which gained to Enoch the reputation of walking with God. "By faith Enoch was translated that he should not see death, and was not found because God had translated him: for before his translation he had this testimony that he pleased God: but without faith it is impossible to please him."

I am to show the consequences of walking with God.

1. By thus walking with God the soul contracts a holy intimacy with him. The consequence is,

2. That it makes advances in the best of all knowledge, the knowledge of God. An intimate walk with God affords an opportunity to study his character, to see it developed in the free communications he makes, and to listen to his instructions. He is the great instructor of mankind; but his teachings are not extended to those who live estranged from him.

3. This closer inspection and clearer discernment of God, are the most powerful means to sanctify the soul. Views of God are transforming. While "with open face" we behold "as in a glass the glory of the Lord," we "are changed into the same image from glory to glory." Therefore,

4. A sure consequence of such an intimacy between God and the soul is an increased mutual affection. The more the soul knows of God the

more it will love him, and of course the more it will be beloved. What a most tender friendship did Enoch and Enoch's God contract for each other during their intimate communion for three hundred years. If we would enjoy the same blessedness, we must, like Enoch, walk with God.

5. Such an intimacy between God and the soul cannot fail to establish mutual confidence. The more God is seen the more securely can the soul commit the management of all its interests to him, and venture its everlasting all upon the truth of his word. On the other hand the more this confidence is found, the more God can confide in such a soul. He will not trust those to whom he can say, "I know you not;" but of those who are intimate with him and confide in him, he will say, "Surely they are my people, children that will not lie." It is the greatest happiness to feel this confidence in God and to know that he has this confidence in us. If we covet this, let us walk with him.

6. Such an intimacy with God will preserve us from bad company. A man who is walking with an honorable friend, is not likely to be annoyed by disagreeable intruders or to break away after low society. When the soul is in the immediate presence of God, neither sin nor Satan dares to invade; neither the world nor any of its perplexing cares will venture to intrude. Every Christian knows what distressing and dangerous companions these are. If we would avoid them and more fully enjoy the profitable

and delightful society of Enoch's God, we must do as Enoch did.

7. Another consequence of such a close walk with God is that we shall find support under the unavoidable trials of life. When we are in distress, very soothing is the company of a prudent and sympathizing friend, who, from the stores of his knowledge, can suggest subjects of consolation. But how much more blissful the society of God, whose heart is all tenderness, and who can open to the soul the most comforting of all truths. There is no consolation like this. Indeed it is well worth while to be a while in the furnace, for the sake of walking there with One in "the form of the Son of God."

8. Another consequence of walking with God is the enjoyment of his protection. Myriads of enemies and dangers swarm in all the way to heaven; but while God is near he will not suffer them to annoy us. When one of Enoch's spirit hears the thunders at a distance, his refuge is nearer than the danger, and he steps in and is safe. He hides himself where no evil or enemy, though searching for him throughout the world, can find him.

9. Another consequence of walking with God is that we shall always have a faithful monitor at hand, to throw in timely cautions to keep us back from indiscretions and sin or to reclaim us when we have wandered. The conscience of one who walks with God is preserved tender, and God is faithful not to suffer a son who

cleaves to him to err by his side without rebuke. To possess such a monitor is one of the greatest blessings of life. Let those who would enjoy this exalted privilege, take care never to depart from the side of their Savior and their God.

10. Another consequence of walking with God is an enlightened view of his providence and government, a clear discernment of the glories of the heavenly world, and a peaceful assurance of his eternal love. Tell me what happiness is if this is not. What, of all the enjoyments of the world, can be *exalted* happiness compared with this?

11. Another effect of walking with God is a higher enjoyment of ordinary blessings. By the placid love which by this means is kept alive, the mind is put in a frame to enjoy every other comfort. And the gratitude which is thus mingled with the enjoyment of God's gifts renders them all the sweeter.

12. Another effect of walking with God is a greater preparation for usefulness. In proportion as the mind becomes wiser by converse with God and holier by near and transforming views of him, it is fitted for stronger and more persevering and better directed efforts for the happiness of others. In proportion as its faith and benevolent desires are enlarged, its prayers will be mighty for the salvation of men. Its very breath will penetrate their conscience and their heart as no other means can do. And it will throw out upon the world the all commanding majesty

and winning sweetness of a holy example. One such man will have more influence upon the order of society and the salvation of men, than millions who never walked with God.

13. Another consequence of walking with God is a peaceful death. In Enoch's case it was not death, but a triumphant translation. And in every other case, in proportion as a man has walked with God, his end, though he leaves his body behind, is still triumphant, or at least serene. How unspeakable a comfort, when one is struggling with the king of terrors and about to enter on eternal and unchangeable scenes, to have "the full assurance of God's love, peace of conscience, and joy in the Holy Ghost." How much better than to sink under awful fears of eternal wrath, or even under doubts which leave the soul to measure over the dark valley alone. Would you enjoy this triumph or even this serenity in death, you must prepare for it by walking with God.

Finally, another consequence of walking thus closely with God, is an enlarged share of immortal glory. In heaven the blessed inhabitants all walk with God, every day and hour. And they find it no burden but a happiness which they would not exchange for the whole creation. Why was it not then happiness on earth? And yet for an exemplary march in that happy course, millions have found their blessedness eternally increased. The enhanced joy of a single soul for a few hours will outweigh all the pleasures of all the wicked on earth. The time will come when that additional blessedness of a single soul, will have out-measured all the happiness enjoyed on earth from Adam to the conflagration. A little further and it will have exceeded all the happiness enjoyed by saints and angels in heaven before the Day of Judgment. And further still, but imagination faints and turns back from the pursuit, and can only exclaim, How infinite the good resulting from one degree of additional faithfulness.

From the weight of all these reasons for a close walk with God, I hope you are now prepared to give your whole attention while,

I state the prominent means by which such a walk can be kept up.

Humility and faith, as we have already seen, are not means merely, but are involved in the very idea of a walk with God. Without these we cannot approach God, much less walk with him. The same may be said of obedience generally. These in the inquiry are not considered so much in the light of means, as a part of the walk which means are to keep up. And yet *particular acts* of disobedience may be mentioned as things to be avoided and particular acts of faith may be named as means to be employed. The means involve two things, the guarding against what is injurious and the attending to what is useful.

I. The guarding against what is injurious.

1. It is absolutely impossible to preserve the soul in the habit of conversing with God, without avoiding improper conversation with men; not only everything false or impure or profane or malicious or revengeful or passionate, but everything deceitful or slanderous or uncharitable or uncandid or vain. It is even

said "that every *idle* word that men shall speak, they shall give account thereof in the day of judgment. For by thy words thou shalt be justified, and by thy words thou shalt be condemned."

2. Vain thoughts are another hindrance to an intimate walk with God. This led the pious Psalmist to say, "I hate vain thoughts." There cannot exist a great degree of spirituality, unless the mind is habitually employed in spiritual contemplations. People, who consume most of their leisure hours in thoughts of vanity, do not walk with God. It betrays a heart full of idolatry: and as well might the worshippers of Baal claim to walk with Israel's God. These cold thoughts diffuse chills of death through all the soul, and can no more coexist with its spiritual activity, than paralysis can coexist with the activity of the body.

3. No known sin must be indulged. One such Achan fostered in our camp, will prove that we have not only no intimacy with God, but no acquaintance with him. One indulged sin is as decisive against us as a hundred. "Whosoever shall keep the whole law and yet offend in one point, he is guilty of all."

4. Undue worldly affections and cares must be excluded. Those affections for the world are undue which are not constantly subjected to the love of God; that is, are not ready, at all times, cheerfully to submit to the rules which he has made to regulate our use and management

of the world, and to any sacrifices which his providence may extort from us or require at our hands. And those cares are undue which, from their number or pressure, seduce the heart from God. Every worldly care necessarily draws the *attention* from God for a season, as we cannot fixedly attend to two things at once. But if the *heart is* not enticed away, the thoughts and affections will spontaneously return to him at every interval of care and with ever fresh delight. Those affections and cares which, according to these definitions, are undue obstruct our communion with God and abate our intimacy with him. Of course they must be guarded against if we would walk with him. These are the things to be studiously avoided. And now,

2. Let us see to what we must attend.

1. We must punctually and earnestly attend on all the means and ordinances of God's appointment. Any neglect or irregularity or carelessness in this attendance, will cut the sinews of our spirituality, and diminish our strength to achieve victories and resist temptations in the future. Separate yourselves from means, and you may as well separate your fields from culture, and even from the rain and dews of heaven. All our light and grace come through the medium of means. This in general; but to be more particular,

2. We must pray the prayer of faith and "pray

without ceasing." Prayer is the Christian's life. Though every other ordinance is attended to, yet if this one be neglected, all is in vain. It is as impossible for the soul to be spiritually alive and active without a punctual course of fervent and believing prayer, as for the body to be alive and active without breath. Prayer has more influence on the sanctification of the soul than all other ordinances. It is going directly to God to receive the life-giving Spirit according to an absolute and often repeated promise. "Ask, and it shall be given to you; seek, and ye shall find; knock, and it shall be opened unto you. For every one that asketh receiveth, and he that seeketh findeth, and to him that knocketh it shall be opened. If a son shall ask bread of any of you that is a father, will he give him astone? or if he ask a fish, will he for a fish give him a serpent? or if he shall ask an egg, will he offer him a scorpion? If ye then, being evil, know how to give good gifts unto your children, how much more shall your heavenly Father give the holy Spirit to them that ask him" Matthew7:7-11.

This is decisive if any language can be. The promise is absolute, and there must be an unwavering belief in the promise in order to give the application success. "If any of you lack wisdom let him ask of God, that giveth to all men liberally and upbraideth not, and it shall be given him. But let him ask in faith, nothing wavering; for he that wavereth is like a wave of the sea driven with the wind and tossed. For let not that man thinks that he shall receive anything of the Lord." But the faith instilled is not a belief that I shall receive, but that I shall receive if I ask aright. It is not a belief in my goodness, but in God's truth. It is a firm, unwavering, confident belief that God will "give the Holy Spirit to them that ask him" *aright*. This strong confidence in God's truth may be exercised whatever doubts we have of our own goodness or election.

If we are troubled on these points it ought not to keep us back. We may leave them to be decided afterwards, and go right to God with unlimited confidence in his truth and consequent willingness to hear the cries of all who sincerely seek him. Whoever is elected, this is true of all. Say not, God will hear me if I am elected, and not without. Election or no election, he certainly will hear the cries of all, (be it Judas or be it Peter,) who seek him with the whole heart. This ought to be the strong confidence of every man, whatever opinion he may have of his own character or destiny. This, as the apostle testifies was the faith of Enoch. "Before his translation he had this testimony that he pleased God. But without faith it is impossible to please him: for he that cometh to God must believe [what? that he himself is good? that he himself is elected? no such thing: must believe] that he is, and that he is a rewarder of them that diligently seek him." There is a full chance then for doubting Christians to exercise this sweet and successful confidence in God.

Tell it to the nations. Let the joyful tidings circulate, through all the region of despondency and gloom. There is no confidence required of you respecting your goodness or election. The only faith demanded is to "believe" in God, "that he is, and that he is a rewarder of them that diligently seek him," whoever they are, whether it is I or another man, elect or non-elect.

3. We must watch. In that most trying moment when the powers of hell were let loose upon the

suffering Savior, he gave his disciples no other direction than this, "Watch and pray that ye enter not into temptation." So much emphasis did he lay on these two duties. In regard to watchfulness, I would suggest the following rules.

First, be vigilant to observe the first motions of the enemy. If he has made considerable advances before you move, your exertions will probably be too late. It is dangerous to parley with temptation. Check it early or it will probably prevail. Keep your eyes open to watch the different avenues by which the enemy makes his approach. He will often vary his mode of attack. Through all his variations keep your eye steadfastly upon him. Acquaint yourselves with his numerous devices.

Secondly, watch another enemy greater than this; watch your own heart. Keep an attentive eye upon the movements of corruption within you: otherwise some evils will gather too much strength for you to resist; others will work unseen, and go in to form your character unknown to yourselves. "Keep thy heart with all diligence, for out of it are the issues of life."Proverbs 4:23.

Thirdly, watch opportunities for doing and getting good. Much is lost in reference to both by overlooking the favorable moment.

Fourthly, watch the motions and expressions of divine providence. It will throw much interesting light on the character and government of God and illustrate and confirm many things taught in the Scriptures.

Fifthly, watch the motions of the Spirit upon your minds. Sometimes the Spirit whispers an invitation to prayer or divine contemplation. If the suggestion is followed we may find the duties easy and pleasant, and the effect lasting. But perhaps we refuse to attend to the impulse. The consequence is, our hearts grow cold and lifeless; and then though we attempt to pray or meditate, we find no relish for it. This remark goes no part of the way towards denying God's efficiency, but only assumes that he leaves us sometimes by way of punishment. It may be illustrated by a passage from the Song of Solomon, understood to relate to the intercourse between Christ and the Church. The Spouse, half aroused from lethargy, says, "I sleep, but my heart waketh: it is the voice of my Beloved that knocketh, saying, Open to me, my sister, my love, my dove, my undefiled; for my head is filled with dew and my locks with the drops of the night. [Now mark how her indolence pleads.] I have put off my coat, how shall I put it on? I have washed my feet, how shall I defile them?

My Beloved put in his hand by the hole of the door, and my bowels were moved for him. I rose up to open to my beloved, end my hands dropped with myrrh, and my fingers with sweet smelling myrrh, upon the handles of the lock. I opened to my Beloved, but, [see the effect of not opening to Christ at first] my Beloved had withdrawn himself and was gone: my soul failed when he spoke: I sought him, but I could not find him; I called him but he gave me no answer."

This is enough to confirm my idea of watching and obeying the first suggestion of the Spirit of

Christ. I have thus shown what it is to walk with God, the blessed consequences, and the means. May I not now, my Christian brethren, urge upon you this delightful duty? It is what you owe to the blessed God, your Father and

Savior, who has astonished heaven by his kindness to you, and whose mercies, if you are not deceived, will hold you entranced to eternity. It is what you owe to him, and it will secure you a happy life, more than all the wealth and honors of the world. It is heaven begun below.

Do you not wish to be happy? Bend all your cares then to walk with God. Be not satisfied with *a general desire* to do this, but fix systematically on the means prescribed. Pursue those means hourly, daily, yearly. Reduce your life to a system under the regulation of these rules. Good old Enoch could walk with God three hundred years. And he has never seen cause to repent it. Could you have access to him in his glory, would he express regret for the pleasant mode of spending the last three hundred years of his life?

We are apt to think that we are not expected to aim at the superior piety of the ancient saints. But why paralyze every power by such a stupid mistake? Are we not under as great obligations? Is not God as worthy of obedience now as in the days of old? Have the increased displays of his mercy in the Gospel impaired his claims? Has the affecting scene of Calvary rendered him less lovely in the eyes of sinners? Are the means used with mankind less than in the patriarchal age? Or are the happy consequences of a walk with God worn out by time? Why should we then content ourselves with being scarcely alive, when so many saints have been through life rapt in communion with God?

Do we thirst for honors? What honor is so great as to be the companion and son and favorite of the everlasting God? Do we wish for riches? Who is as rich as the heir of him who owns all the treasures of the universe? Do we prize the best society? What better society can be found than Enoch had? Does any valuable consideration move us, or any ingenuous motive, O let us never cease to walk with God. Leaders are born as well prepared and guided into maintaining their potentials as servants and pillars in the house of God.

The mark of the dynamic leader is clearly manifested in whatever he puts his hand to. It is therefore, my hope that Christian leaders will devote their priorities to gain a place for the church in the focus point in society. A spirit of adventure; the urge to explore and real new grounds, challenge the status quo, stand up for what you believe, something you think is worth saying to improve the world around you. Have the courage to peak out and the willingness to risk group rejection. You can modify your style of influencing a bit, bit but not totally.

A quietly persuasive leader wills you must bear the fruits of the spirit. By doing thus it will allow you to resist the flesh or anything that may hinder your spirit. Your spirit must be like that candle that giveth light continually. He wrote the Epistle that those who believe might know they have eternal life (John 8:32) and he shall know the truth, and the truth shall make you free. This in means you must believe the truth of God's word as it is revealed in His word and that makes a sincere and sustained effort by His grace to follow it in word and deed.

The blood of Jesus Christ, His son cleansed us from all of our sins. It refers to the ongoing work of sanctification within believers and continually cleansing through the blood of Christ of our inadvertent sin. Of walking in the light (1 John 1:7) it is continuous cleansing that allows us to have an intimate fellowship with God.

We must be holy, and consecrated, and separated from the world. In order to live this life we must love God with all our hearts, soul, mind, and body. God's children achieve sanctification by faith and union with Christ in His death and resurrection by the blood of Christ and by the working of the Holy Spirit.

Chapter Seven

Are We Spirit Filled Believers?

Spirit filled believers are tested daily. "*My brethren, count it all joy when ye fall into divers temptations; 3 knowing this, that the trying of your faith worketh patience. 4 But let patience have her perfect work, that ye may be perfect and entire, wanting nothing*" (James 1: 2-4).

Testing is part of the believers walk with God. We should count it a glorious opportunity of proving our faith. Consider it pure joy because of what trials can produce in our lives. James tells us to turn our hardships into times of learning. Tough times can teach us perseverance. We can't really know the depth of our character until we see and react under pressure.

"*The joy of the Lord is your strength*" (Philippians 1:4). Always in every prayer be sure to make your request with joy. "*And having this confidence, I know that I shall abide and continue with you all for your furtherance and joy of faith*" (Philippians 1:25).

Patience is more necessary than anything else in our faith walk. Timing with God is nothing; for a thousand years is as one day and a day is a thousand years. Christ's purpose in our lives is that we should be perfect and wanting nothing. James 1: 12-14 says *"Blessed is the man that endureth temptation: for when he is tried, he shall receive the crown of life, which the Lord hath promised to them that love him. Let no man say when he is tempted, I am tempted of God: for God cannot be tempted with evil, neither tempteth he any man: but every man is tempted, when he is drawn away of his own lust, and enticed."*

Temptation

Temptation basically comes from our inward desire where our inclination or evil desire is not resisted and despite purges by the Holy Spirit, it leads to sin and then spiritual death. No person, who sins can invade guilt by throwing the blame on God. God test us in order to strengthen our faith but never is the intention of leading us to sin. The nature of God demonstrates that He cannot be the source of temptation. Temptation does not refer to enticement to sin, but to trials, persecution and afflictions from the world of Satan.

The believers must meet these trials with joy, for they will develop patience (i.e., perseverance, endurance). Our faith can only reach full maturity when faced with difficulties and oppositions. James called these trials a *"trying of your faith."*

Trials are sometimes brought into a believer's life so that God can test their faith. Scripture nowhere teaches that troubles in life are always an indication that God is displeased with us.

Our very thoughts can lead us into temptation; that is why Apostle Paul said in Philippians 4:8: "***whatsoever things are true, whatsoever things are honest, whatsoever things are just, whatsoever things are pure, whatsoever things are lovely, whatsoever things are of good report; if there be any virtue, and if there be any praise, think on these things.***"

It can be a sign that He recognized our firm commitment to Him.

Chapter Eight

$\mathcal{A}$ $\mathcal{C}$ommitted $\mathcal{L}$eader

The vision aims to form leaders with cultures of the kingdoms that is, people who are able to influence others, and together will make up the basis growth for the church. For example there was a point in time when I sought the Lord concerning ministry and who He wanted to be my leaders in ministry. A couple of days later I was praying when the Lord said to me "You must walk down the road." But what I did not know was that He was leading me to someone who is my song leader and his family house.

God has set me up with this family to fulfill the work that He called me to do. This family has been a big influence in my life where ministry is concerned. We also received a musician out of this family that God has given us.

These are leaders with a spirit of servitude, who will become the successors of the generations to come so that the word of God continues. These are the kinds of leaders formed through the vision. The importance of the vision is that people will perish without a vision. Imposing the vision oneself by living first in order to pass it on afterwards. We started to unit together as a ream working to meet the need of the community. One of the first things that I believe the ministry is called to be is a strong foundation by God.

The Church is called to Evangelize

The first purpose for which the church was called was to evangelize the earth (Matthew 28: 19-20). When we lose sight of this calling, we become cultish in our desire to keep things of God for ourselves.

- We are appointed as watchman on the walls to warm the world of the consequences of their sinful behavior. (Ezekiel 33: 1-9). We are responsible to others about the saving grace available through Jesus Christ. If we fail to remember this then we are liable before.

- The pattern for evangelism is established in the Scripture (Acts 1:8). Our first obligation is to our families. This is our Jerusalem. Once we have taken care of our own household, then we are ready to move on.

- Jerusalem - is my house.

- Judah - is my neighborhood

- Samaria - is my city.

- The uttermost part of the world.

The Church is called to Edify

The second purpose for which the church was created was

to bring edification or maturity to the disciples of Christ (Ephesians 4: 11-16). God has called us to win the lost and then to build them up in Him. Going to Bible School is my training in the Word of God and it is the most important aspect of this function. When we know the word we are less susceptible to false teaching. Paul would trust that Timothy had been built up by the word substantially enough to confront false doctrines that were circulating. (Philippians 2: 12 - 18).

As the Christ lives in the church, the nature of Christ should be apparently within the church. The people of God are able to reflect the Holiness of God. (Romans 12:12). The church has a special relationship to the Lord because we have been consecrated into His service. While sewing in the basement; the Lord appeared to me and confirmed that the calling of my life is to feed his sheep (John 21:15-16) as He repairs broken lives through Healing Waters Ministry.

I was faces many times with challenges from my peers; it allowed me to think an even question myself. I was called for ministry, and every time it crossed my mind God will have someone to encourage me about what God has called me to do. My confidence will always be building for the good and tearing down the bad. In obedience to God's plan and purpose for my life, I had to win the ultimate battle.

Love's Thou Me

The most important question that Peter ever faces was whether possessed a devoted love for His Lord. There are two Greek words for "love" used here. The first "agape" which means an intelligent and purposeful love, primarily of mind and will. The second "phileo" which means to involve warm natural affection of the emotions, thus a more personal and feeling love.

Through these two words, Jesus indicated that Peter's love must be not only if the will, but also of the heart, a love springing from both purpose and personal attachment. We must all have a personal heartfelt love and devotion to Jesus (John 14:15). Jesus considered love for him as the basic qualifications for Christian service. Other qualifications are needed (1 Tim 3:1-13) but love for Christ and others are indispensable (1 Cor. 13:1-3). Stir up the unused gifts in the body of Christ. The bible says that we must stir up the gifts that are in them as fire under the embers. He must take all opportunities to use these gifs, for that is the best way to increase them. The great hindrance of usefulness is in the increase of our gifts in slavish fear.

Paul therefore warns Timothy this (2 Timothy 1:7) God had delivered us from the spirit of fear, and given us power, love and a sound mind. The spirit of power or of courage and resolution, the spirit of love to God which will set us above the fear of man, and the spirit of a sound mind, or quietness of a mind for we are often discouraged in our worked with the creatures of our own imagination, which a sober, thinking mind would obliterate.

Feed My Sheep

One day I was seeking the face of the Lord, He told me to feed His sheep on many occasions. The Lord would be speaking to me to feed my sheep. I was a sheep myself so the thought of me feeding sheep was very astonishing. We can have our lives all planned out and God may have another plan for our lives. Preaching the Word of God was never a thought that was in my mind. Believe it or not everyone has a calling on his/her life and many of us are running from our call. As I hear many people give testimonies about their calling I fell as though I fall into the same category. Jesus description of believers as lambs and sheep implies three things.

1.   We need continual pastoral care

2.   We are to feed constantly upon the Word of God

3.   Since the sheep are prone to wander into danger, we need repeated guidance, protection, and correction.

It is good when you are guided by the Lord. He will be faithful with believers in His wisdom concerning this guidance, note the following truths.

1.   God has a plan for every believer; He had a plan for Adam (Genesis 1:8) God placed them in the Garden of Eden and gave them dominion over the earth. Everything belonged to them. God made full provision to meet all their needs. God began his relationship with man through an acting giving. He placed them in a beautiful garden and gave them herbs and fruit bearing trees for their food. They had everything that they needed. God gave them the entire world with all its recourses.

As I waited in His presence He would reveal many things to me about His people. The Lord gave me many dreams about the future; some I couldn't understand until they actual became fulfilled. I wrote many of the dreams down, so that I could remember them as they were coming into manifestation. There were many times that I had an angelic visit from the angels in heaven and they caused me to become afraid.

One morning I was awaken by an audible voice to go into the entire world and lay hands on the sick and they shall recover, which led to (Mark 16:18) The scriptures clearly teach that it is desire of Christ for His followers to perform miraculous deeds as they announce the gospel of the Kingdom of God (Matt. 10:1) Theses are the signs performed by the disciples, confirm that the gospel message is genuine that the Kingdom of God has come to earth in power and the living and risen Jesus is present with His people and working through them (Acts 10:38) How God anointed Jesus of Nazareth with the Holy Ghost and with power; Who went about doing and healing all that were oppressed of the devil for God was with him.

- Every one of these signs occurred in the recorded history of the church.
- Speaking in tongues
- Expelling demons
- Escaping death from snake bites and healing the sick

These spiritual manifestations are intended to continue within Christian churches until Jesus returns. These scriptures never suggest that signs were restricted to the period immediately following ascension (1 Cor. 1:7, 12:28)

It's clear that the followers of Christ were to preach the gospel of the Kingdom and bring salvation to those who believe (Matt 28:19-20) but were also to bring in that kingdom just as Jesus did by casting demons and healing diseases, and sickness (Acts 10:38) Jesus indicates in Mark 16:15-20, these signs are not special gifts for a few but were to be given to all believers who in obedience to Christ, witness to the gospel and claimed His promises. Jesus promised that His authority, power, and presence would accompany us as we battle the kingdom of Satan. We must liberate people from their captivity by preaching the gospel, by living a righteous life and by performing signs and miracles through the power of the Holy Spirit (Mark 16:16-20).I could remember about twenty three years ago, the clock struck at four in the morning and the Lord gave me a visit in my bedroom. I was awakening from out of a dream with a voice calling me it said "daughter, go in all the world and lay hands on the sick in my name and they shall be delivered." It felt as though someone was holding my right hand and it was hot as if it had just come out of the oven. It would occur many times after this morning. On several occasions I had visitations where I told someone something, and they would think that I am out of my mind. From the day the Lord saved me there had been many prophecies over my life. But, dying was not one of them. I believe in speaking Gods word over my life daily for my protection.

Chapter Nine

The Birth of the Ministry

He also spoke the word and life came into existence, a person who is a carrier of the Word of God. As Healing Waters Ministry started I promised myself that it would be everything the Lord said that it will be. The vision of the Holy Waters would rise and extend in depth of healing virtue, the fish in them (the fish meaning people) and an account of the trees growing on the banks (Ezekiel 47:1-12) The vision has a mystical and a spiritual meaning.

The prophecy, explained in (Zechariah 14:1-12). Living waters shall go from Jerusalem, half of them towards the corner sea and half towards the hinder sea. That seems to represent grace and joy where glory began. Most interpreters agree that these waters signify the gospel of Christ, which went from Jerusalem and spread itself into other countries and the gifts and powers of the Holy Ghost which accompany it. By virtue of which it spreads far and produces blessed effects. This is the spirit of God that was poured out on the apostles and embedded with the power to go forth and preach the gospel to all nations, heal the sick, cast out devils, raise the dead; freely they received and freely give. It believes in Him that we receive from the rivers of living waters, and he spoke of the Spirit in John 7:38-39.

I believe the Healing waters Ministry will be a ministry that will spread from the community to all parts of the world.

As I read the scriptures in the book Ezekiel 47:1-12 it started off the house westward, meaning ankle deep was the starting point and from that point it goes to knee into deeper revelation in intercession, the prophet not only was present but he was the future, under the right side of the house, that is, the south side of the altar, this is why I could understand that this ministry takes a lot of warfare and a lot of praying. Our services were being held at two in the evening.

But one day there was an elderly lady who came to worship with us. As I was delivering the Word of God to His people. God gave me a word concerning some of the future matters that were going to take place. The scripture says that with man it is impossible, but with God all things are possible. You have to tell yourself that you are more than a conqueror and that you are on this earth for a purpose. And everything that is not of God has to be removed.

Spiritual Warfare

Our life is engaged in warfare because we struggle with common calamities of human life. We struggle with opposition of the power of darkness and wickedness in high places. Paul the apostle wrote to the church in the book of Ephesians 6:10: "*be strong in the Lord, and in the power of his might,*" meaning to equip yourself like men and fight like a man with the power that is within you. God is the one that is fighting for you and not you, yourself.

As a Christian, we engage in a spiritual conflict with evil. This spiritual conflict is described as warfare of faith as recorded in 2 Corinthians 10:4: "*for the weapons of our warfare are not carnal, but mighty through God to the pulling down of strong holds.*" Also, 2 Timothy 2: 18-19: "*who concerning the truth have erred, saying that the resurrection is past already; and overthrow the faith of some. 19 Nevertheless the foundation of God standeth sure, having this seal, The Lord knoweth them that are his. And, Let every one that nameth the name of Christ depart from iniquity.*"

We have received our marching orders to advance into Satan's territory and take back what Satan has stolen from us. When you think of what God's Word has said, we are not defeated nor are we on the defensive as we are no longer running afraid. But we are pressing into battle, going to wage offensive war to win, know that Christ set us free from the power of sin; and He has restored the control of our will so that we can take power of sin, and the ability to bring every thought under control of the Holy Spirit, bring our will into submission to God's will.

Nothing can every stop a believer's victory when he or she knows that they have been secured by Christ Himself through His death on the cross. Jesus waged a triumphant battle against Satan's domain. In Paul writing to the church as recorded in 2 Timothy 4: 7-8: "*I have fought a good fight, I have finished my course, I have kept the faith: 8 henceforth there is laid up for me a crown of righteousness, which the Lord, the righteous judge, shall*

give me at that day: and not to me only, but unto all them also that love his appearing."

At this present time Christians are involved in spiritual warfare that they wage by the power of the Holy Spirit against the corrupt desire within themselves. Romans 8:13 says: "***For if ye live after the flesh, ye shall die: but if ye through the Spirit do mortify the deeds of the body, ye shall live.***" There are ungodly pleasures of this work and temptation of every sort. Matthew 13:22 says: "***He also that received seed among the thorns is he that heareth the word; and the care of this world, and the deceitfulness of riches, choke the word, and he becometh unfruitful.***"

You Must Be Pure

"***Who shall ascend into the hill of the Lord? Or who shall stand in his holy place?***

He that hath clean hands, and a pure heart; who hath not lifted up his soul unto vanity, nor sworn deceitfully.

He shall receive the blessing from the Lord, and righteousness from the God of his salvation. (Psalm 24: 3-5)."

Our hearts must be right. For our own good we must cultivate new seeds God has placed in our hearts, He will plant seeds in your heart that will produce fruit until Jesus comes.

There are measures to take, nothing comes easy and spiritual fruit will not come automatically. None of the manifestations of God's power and blessings are going to come automatically down from heaven in your life. God seeds and His planting contain the ability to produce spiritual fruit, but the growth of that seed will depend on you. There are some things you must bear in mind before the seed of revelation, love, faith and power can germinate, grow and produce fruit in your life. Certain conditions must be met:

1. They must be sown in fertile soil (meaning your heart).

2. They must receive proper care and nourishment.

Unless these conditions are met, the spiritual seeds will remain dormant and unproductive in your life. The ability to produce spiritual fruit is still in the seed and for it to grow these conditions must be met. It takes spiritual energy. In other words you have to press your way through. Many times you will be drained. One of the secrets I found is to separate myself from the present world system - on hating all its evil and overcoming and dying to its temptation and condemnation and condemning open sin.

Hebrew 1:9 tells us that Christian soldiers must wage war against all evil, not in their own power, but with spiritual weapons. In their warfare of faith, Christians care called upon to endure hardship as good soldiers of Christ and to suffer for the gospel. Matthew 5: 10-12 says: "***Blessed are they which are persecuted for righteousness' sake: for theirs is the kingdom of heaven.***

Blessed are ye, when men shall revile you, and persecute you, and shall say all manner of evil against you falsely, for my sake. Rejoice, and be exceeding glad: for great is your reward in heaven: for so persecuted they the prophets which were before you." Also Romans 8:17 says: "***and if children, then heirs; heirs of God, and joint-heirs***

with Christ; if so be that we suffer with him, that we may be also glorified together."

You must determine and claim the spiritual territory that legally belongs to you through Christ. If you do not know then you give the enemy your legal rights. God has not planned any defeat for you.

Approximately three years ago, I was at a prayer meeting and the some of the prayer warriors were at my side and they were praying for the Lord to heal me. I had prayed for so many people with different sickness and they had gotten healed. Also, I could remember the previous illnesses that the Lord had healed me from. There are even scars to prove it. Take for instance, my youngest daughter. She was born with her skin looking like an old lady because of the difficulties that I had during the pregnancy and God performed a miracle on her body.

Next my granddaughter was born and it seemed that everything that could go wrong went wrong. Again the miraculous hand of Jesus came to help us through. Many times she would actually expire (die), but we prayed and God heard and answered our prayers for her to live again.

I understand what pray can do. And no one told me that the road would be easy. Though these times of suffering I learned how to fight the good fight of faith. I waged war, persevered, conquered, was victorious, and I defended the gospel and continue to strive toward my goals. My faith was high and I could truly say that 'God was on my side' because I learned to put my trust totally in Him.

The Scriptures states clearly and simply that faith comes by hearing and hearing by the Word of God. God word is two things: it is **written word** and it is the **living** word. You have

God's faith when His living word is living on the inside of you. The living word never changes, for it is eternal.

It has no beginning and it has no ending; it is God Himself. You cannot separate God from His word for God and His Word are one.

In the New Testament three are two Greek words which are translated into "word." While both of these expressions mean "word" each has its own specific distinct meaning. One of these Greek words is "logos" and the other is "Rhema." The "logos means what goes beyond the spoken and the written word. The Greek Lexicon tells us that it gives a depth of meaning far beyond that which is written and that which is spoken. Actually, it denotes an extension and an expression of that which comes not from the lips or from the pen, but that which comes from the mind. It is in the mind where the concept of thought and the concept of intelligence begin.

The word "Logos" gives us the understanding of what goes beyond the spoken or written word. It is implied to us by the Holy Spirit that this is something that is self-existent. In other words, it has no beginning of days and it has no end of life. It is a being that stands all by itself. The logos is that self-existent power we know to be the word Himself, they living word, Christ.

"Rhema" is a word from God which is an extension of the Logos and it is not the spoken or written word that comes to us out of the suggestions of the mind of God. "Rhema" is derived from a verb and it means "action" "to speak" or to speak a word Rhema comes from the very strength of the Logos Himself.

As the Rhema is the spoken word, this Logos is the express of the Logos that the word is formed that comes to us from the Rhema. When we receive it, we are receiving the words of man but we are speaking the thoughts of God.

There are many people who feel very weak, as if they have no faith at all. But you must strive for the faith and not be alarmed by your components. I put on the full armor of God. Stand firm to destroy Satan's strongholds and take captive every thought. Become mighty in war, and content in the faith. Lay hold of eternal life.

Many things have developed out of my home, family, children and ministry. Such as many marriages that were healed. Many people got delivered from demonic stronghold. I was travelling to different places and ministering to God's people . . . it was a joy in my heart to do so.

God has seasoned me with grace and made me stronger in my life. I have come to the understanding that God was processing me for a great and more effective life. Faith in Jesus Christ is the only condition that God requires for salvation. Faith is not only a profession about Christ, but also an activity coming from the heart of believers who seeks to follow Christ as Lord and Savior. (Matthew 4: 19; John 10: 4, 27). The conception of faith includes two elements:

1. Faith means firmly believing and trusting in the crucified and risen Christ as our Lord and Savior. It involves believing from the heart. That is yielding up our will and committing our total selves to Jesus Christ as he revealed in the New Testament.

2. Faith involves repentance. Turning away from sin with true sorrow and turning to God through Christ. Saving faith is away a repentant faith.

Faith is the ultimate sense that cannot properly be distinguished from love. How do people see you? It is by the love you show one another, someone asked the question "what is the difference between you and others?" My answer is 'the love of God makes the difference. I don't know anything else." It is a personal activity of sacrifice and self-giving directed toward Christ (Matt. 22:37; John 21: 15-17).

The Heart of Pastors

Always love to provoke people to worship the Lord. That is the most important part of the service where I see the manifested power of the Holy Spirit that touches lives in the services and the people are changed from glory to glory. As our worship leader would take the people into the presence of the Lord things would happen.

The book of Revelation describes worship experience in heaven. And as the saints worship, God was the object of their affection and worship. When we give praise to the Lamb of God, we offer worship that is pleasing, that is appropriate and pleasing to the Father. Unless our worship centers on the person and the work of Jesus Christ it is not appropriate. Because of Jesus' obedience to the Father, He has been the object of all worship. (Philippians 2: 9-11).

We worship Christ because He alone achieved our redemption. The access we have to God is gained only through the sacrifice of our loving Savior. We are only acceptable to God because of the intercession of Christ as recorded in Revelation 5: 9-10.

Through my times of healing, worship became the center

of my life and still is. We worship Christ because He has restored the inheritance that was lost due to sin. Jesus is a worthy object of our worship because He has returned what the enemy of our souls sought to steal. Through His ministry, we once again experience paradise. Meaning everyone sometime or another should have an experience of that presence for themselves.

In the year of 2007, I just had to give God something special as we gathered at the church where I attended and we were having a praise rally. The presence of the Lord was so real and I just knew that the Lord was pleased as I was so happy that He had manifested His presence in our midst.

Worship purifies us and brings us closer to the image of Christ. In Isaiah 6: 1-7, you will see that Isaiah came into the presence of the Lord. And as he worshipped he realized his sinful state. God provided a purging of this sinful nature as he was worshipping with God.

Leaders in the Church

As a leader of Healing Waters Ministry, I see great potential in the people that God sent our way. I encourage the people to be dedicated to the Lord and to what God has called them to do. The gifts and talents among our young people have already begun to manifest and they have started to utilize their gift as they develop their maturity in the Lord.

All they needed was to be encouraged to submit to the will of God, and give God the talents that He had given them, for God chose them for such a time as this. That is why I can look back and see the hand of the Lord in all that I have been through and still say 'to God be the glory for the things He has done.' Many other have gone through the same thing I have, but they never made it through, for many died along the way.

Every leader goes through things in their lives give them a testimony, and what they go through many times changes everything about them.

There is a definite structure to the leadership in the church. God has appointed particular offices in the body of Christ. These offices have specific functions. Each of these offices should be exercised in the church today. **Apostles** are those who are sent out to begin churches. 1 Corinthians 9: 1-2 says: "*Am I not an apostle? Am I not free? Have I not seen Jesus Christ our Lord? Are not ye my work in the Lord? If I be not an apostle unto others, yet doubtless I am to you: for the seal of mine apostleship are ye in the Lord.*"

Paul's authority was questioned by some of the Corinthians of his rights as an apostle. He gave his credentials and told them that he actually talked with Christ who had called him to be an apostle. Such credentials make the advice he gives in the letters more persuasive. 2 Corinthians 10:13 says: "*But we will not boast of things without our measure, but according to the measure of the rule which God hath distributed to us, a measure to reach even unto you.*" Paul defends his apostleship in greater detail. His life was changed and there was evidence that God was using him.

Does your life or your faith have an impact on others? You can be a life changer, helping others grow spiritually if you dedicate yourself to be used by God and let Him make you effective. Paul also gave an illustration of giving up his personal rights; he had the right to hospitality, the right to be married, and to be paid for his work. But he willingly gave up these rights to win people to Christ. When your focus is on living for Christ, your rights become unimportant.

Then you have the **prophets.** Those who are called to bring a message of discipline and repentance to the church (Acts 5: 1-11). We see that both external and internal problems were facing the church. Inside the church were honesty and administrative headaches and outside the church was there persecution. As a leader, you have to be careful and sensitive in knowing how to deal with internal matters. You can't avoid external pressure and through it all, the leaders have to keep their focus on what is most important and that is spreading the good news of Jesus.

The *evangelists* are those who are gifted in presenting the gospel and leading others to Christ (Acts 8: 26-36). It's like Philip who was having success preaching to great crowds in Samaria. There will be times where you might understand everything, you just have to be sensitive and follow the leading of the Lord.

Nothing comes easy. You must let God lead your ministry Pastors are those who are appointed to shepherd the flock. This is a resident ministry where as the previous three are most frequently seen in Scripture as itinerate. The pastors are the stewards for the flock under God's authority.

Teachers are those who are gifted to present the doctrine of faith consistent with the Word of God. Just as one of the leaders can have all the leadership gifts residing in him/her; God uses many people to display His works and bring unity from diversity.

The goal of the church's leadership is to bring people into maturity in Christ. As the leaders fill their function, the members become more like Christ and are therefore growing into a Holy Nation unto Him. The result is unity of the body.

The ministry is still young and I am only taking baby steps as I go along and as the Lord leads and directs me on this journey. I will lead to the best of my ability and with the Holy Spirit on leading me, I can't go wrong. I believe the nations can be affect by what God is saying to you to do.

I was told by a man of God that I was destines for greater favor. Psalm 71:21 says: "*Thou shalt increase my greatness, and comfort me on every side*." One of the things he said is that greatness starts with me. God is removing from my life all the distractions and people who mean me harm in this season. Don't allow non-achievers to stand in your way. Don't be afraid to let them go; the only thing standing between you and greatness is you. Apostle Paul has a revelation of God's Word that all true revelation is to bring us into a deeper knowledge of Christ Himself and the life within us; also to draw us into greater knowledge and experience of God through His Son, Jesus Christ.

The definition of **Revelations** is the drawing of the veil of darkness between you and God. You have to be separated where it is God and you. You have to learn to take steps toward your greatness. What are you doing with your life? What is the point of trying to make do and live in mediocrity, fear and confusion. Personal greatness is a choice and we even get to choose what it means to us.

Greatness is found walking down the corridor of your uniqueness. And to realize that greatness, it is necessary to smash through the door of conformity. Standing at the threshold of that door is when you feel your greatest fears. It is often ourselves that keeps us from embracing our uniqueness and realizing our greatness. You have to press your way through for greater success. One morning at 4:00 am, I was awakened by a presence at the foot of my bed. I saw a white eagle at the foot of my bed. The revelation that came from that is that God is about to elevate my life to another level.

Chapter Ten

Delayed But Not Forgotten

When a person is delayed it does not mean that they are forgotten. It is only for a little while. Things don't come to you easy. Some things are delayed for the right timing. Your time and God's time is totally different. Because God knows what is best for you. Often times He will test you to see what you can handle. Many times the situation and circumstances of trials that surrounds you only makes you strong and wiser. You get a little more knowledge and understanding.

Some of the times we carry poor judgment on our part. Jesus called the twelve disciples and everyone has their assignment to carry out. Just as He called the church and gave them their assignment to carry out, just as He called the church and gave them their assignment to go out in all the world and preach the good news to the poor. He sent me to heal the broken hearted, to preach deliverance to the captives, recover the sight to the blind, and the set liberty to them that are bruised. To preach the acceptable year of the Lord (Luke 4: 18-19).

There is one problem. We as the people of God don't listen half of the time. If we would walk in our call, many lives would be changed. I can support this statement because I ran from the Lord from the age of thirteen until I was twenty-nine years old. The ministry should be much further along, but my running only delayed it. But I am glad for the delays, because it is like a wilderness experience which even prepares you the more for ministry.

One of the most important strategies Jesus used to defeat Satan was that He was prepared. He was ready at all times to face the enemy. He could not be taken by surprise. Before He began His earthly ministry, before He performed miracles, He was well prepared.

Your knowledge of Christ, your relationship, your union with Him through prayer is the source and foundation of your strength. Unless you are will to discipline your life as Jesus did to include consistent times of prayer with Him, in which you are allowing Him to reveal Himself to you, consistent times of prayer with Him, in which you are allowing Him to reveal Himself to you, you will not be able to survive.

You cannot be taken by surprise if you are fasting and praying and building yourself in the most holy faith. This puts you on the offensive side to defeat the enemy. Every day comes with advantages and disadvantages. How do you see or view your day? Don't worry about the little things that come to distract you, as long as you know that God is with you, then you can greet your days and it will determine what your future will be. No day comes empty, every day comes with fullness. It is with night and day, but you're still in that day. Whatever you do and live in that day is important. It is important to stay focused and it will change your way of thinking. A man of God wrote "God does not anoint coward, He anoints warriors."

Jericho is a warfare place of power where you stay until you can break through for victory. Gilgal is a place of faith that brings you to the place of power and you stay there no matter what. When God gives you a word, don't let it go. When God told me that He had a set time for my healing, I had to trust God with everything I had within me. I knew that God has plans for my life and no matter how it looked; I knew that my deliverance was coming.

When my brothers and sisters see me today, they often say to me that it looks as though I had not gone through anything. What I went through for the glory of God. It was not about me, but it was about Jesus. What can we offer our generation if we don't go through anything. My life is a miracle all the way through.

As children of God, if we would understand the kingdom of God, we will find out that it is all about standing on our own feet and taking our place as sons and daughters of God. I learned lately how to understand the kingdom message. It had been taught to me before, but I had never grasped it like I do now.

There I was preaching this message about women of the kingdom when the word went forth and it really impacted these women and it was such a blessing in my sister's church that many of these women were set free by the power of God. I would like to go a little deeper with this. According to the Word of God, the kingdom of God is within you and you have to activate it, and understand your purpose here on this earth.

What is your Purpose?

Your purpose is to do the will of you Father on this earth. It goes back to the Book of Genesis 1:26. Right in the Garden when God made man and gave him dominion over the earth. Dominion in Hebrew is "kingdom." A "kingdom" is the governing influence of a king over a territory. The king impacts the dominion with his will and his purposes so that he can produce people who reflect the king's morals and values. Matthew 25:34 says: "***Then shall the King say unto them on his right hand, Come, ye blessed of my Father, inherit the kingdom prepared for you from the foundation of the world.***"

The Father has an inheritance for me that I haven't tapped into yet. If the kingdom is in me and I am in the kingdom, then I must activate what is necessary for my life without fear and unbelief. Luke 18:1 says "***And he spake a parable unto them to this end, that men ought always to pray, and not to faint.***"

Think for a moment about strongholds Satan has on the lives of others in our homes, our communities and our nations. Many Christians are facing situations and problems that are causing them to be confused and afraid. They don't even know how to pray concerning themselves. Many have been attacked physically and mentally. Their strength seems to be gone and they are discouraged.

Many times as a counselor I have had to seek God for direction in certain cases. I have had many encounters with the enemy while praying and this was my only hope. That's why men must always pray and not faint.

One day after I had finished praying, there was a phone call that came for my husband, but he was not home at that time. And as I answered something happened, because right after I hung up the phone immediately rang again. This person said to me 'could you be my mother?' My answer was 'yes' with no hesitation. I have been a mother to many, but this time it was completely different as if I had given birth to my own child. So the relationship begins to grow. This person calls me at times and we often pray together.

We should commit every fiber of our being to the will of God. When you are in God's will, it is very important to the children of God. I have received many healings in my body on many occasions. God wants His children to be made whole in perfect health. There is no doubt about this: healing is not an option, it is a promise that God made His children.

Some people think that healing is not for today. I dare anyone to think that God is dead. He is alive and still in the healing business. I saw my hands grow out before my own eyes. Once my back was messed up because of an accident, and it caused one of my legs to be longer (by an inch). I was in a revival service and the man of God touched me and my leg grew out one inch to match the other leg.

Another incident that happen was when my third sister was pregnant with her last son, the baby died in her. The doctor told her that she would have to abort the baby. She was four months pregnant at the time. She and I came together in prayer in agreement for the life of the baby and one hour later the baby leaped in her womb. That's a miracle! We give

God praise. My nephew is nineteen years old and looking forward to his destiny. My sister is serving God with a passion and nothing can stop her.

Sometimes the experience that you go through will take you to a place that you don't want anything coming between you and your Savior, and you press no matter what you go through.

Jehovah Tsidkenu, the Lord our Righteousness, you can rest assured that His love for you is certain. It will never change. Destiny is calling our name and God is positioning me to receive what He has in store for me. Psalm 71:21 says: "***Thou shalt increase my greatness, and comfort me on every side.***" Wherever I go people would be talking to me about their lives. The anointing makes a difference that you can touch the lives of others. Whatever you do, let not your past rob you of your rich future.

Sickness

There are two redemptive blessings which Christ brought o the world. They are salvation and healing-deliverance from sin and sickness. Salvation from sin and sickness or healing from sin and sickness are both blessings which is one atonement. It's provided by one sacrifice and by one substitute.

John 8:32 says "***and ye shall know the truth, and the truth shall make you free.***" **e has inHe**This truth sets men free in their bodies as well as their souls. Many of the places that I have had the opportunity to preach God's word would come for salvation and become saved from their sins and not be healed from their sickness. After they heard the truth and believed, they were healed and delivered.

Paul said in 1 Corinthians 6:20 "*For ye are bought with a price: therefore glorify God in your body, and in your spirit, which are God's.*" Peter told the crippled man in Acts 3:6 "*Silver and gold have I none; but such as I have give I thee: In the name of Jesus Christ of Nazareth rise up and walk.*" Paul said to the demon in Acts 16:18 "*I command thee in the name of Jesus Christ to come out of her. And he came out the same hour.*"

Jesus left His name with us. It dwells with us and we have the right to use it. Jesus is saying, "You ask the Father in My name and He will do it." As we take our privileges and rights in the new covenant, and pray in Jesus' name our request, the petition passes out of our hands into the hand of Jesus. He accepts the responsibility of that need, and we know that He said "Father, I thank Thee that Thou hearest me and know that Thou hearest me always." In other words, we know that the Father always hears Jesus and when we pray in Jesus' name, it is as though Jesus Himself was doing the praying . . . He takes our place.

So if you need a healing, you can ask the Father for it in Jesus' name. Believe that He hears you and you will find that your sickness will leave. Why? "*And this is the confidence that we have in him, that, if we ask any thing according to his will, he heareth us: (verse 15) and if we know that he hear us, whatsoever we ask, we know that we have the petitions that we desired of him*" (1 John 5: 14-15).

"*And whatsoever ye shall ask in my name, that will I do, that the Father may be glorified in the Son. If ye shall ask any thing in my name, I will do it*" (John 14: 13-14). Again, you have permission to use His name in prayer. Hebrew 4:12 says "*For the word of God is quick, and powerful, and sharper than any twoedged sword,*"

piercing even to the dividing asunder of soul and spirit, and of the joints and marrow, and is a discerner of the thoughts and intents of the heart. " John 1:1 says: "***In the beginning was the Word, and the Word was with God, and the Word was God.*** "

Just as I am finishing this, I received a word from the prophet saying the very Scripture that I was using at this point in this book. God will always confirm His Word to let you know you are on the right track.

I believe that God wants us to recognize His voice. He wants you to hear Him every day and not just on special occasions. The prophet encourages me to prepare my heart and mind to hear from the Lord. Because once you begin to listen to God, He will speak to you in many ways. The Lord is speaking to me and I thank God for my husband because I had to travel to minister into another State. This also gives me an opportunity to seek the Lord. God also gave me many visions in the book of Ephesians (Ephesians 1: 16-17), and it was distinctly personal. For it is written that eyes have not seen nor ears heard, and what entered into one's own heart of all those things God prepared for them that love Him (I Corinthians 2:9).

These are not the days where God wants his people to be ignorant or for things to remain as a mystery Ephesians 1:18 says: "***the eyes of your understanding being enlightened; that ye may know what is the hope of his calling, and what the riches of the glory of his inheritance in the saints.*** " Paul prayed that revelation would come to the believer's life and that they would come to full understanding of Christ Himself and life within us. And to draw us into a greater knowledge and experience of God's son Jesus Christ.

Full understanding of the spirit of spiritual riches of the Lord is passing us through His operation in others. You will have greater use of the spiritual power He freely gave unto us, the church is afraid to use our spiritual authority. As I studied the book of Ephesians there is a passage in (John 2:17") and His disciples remembered that it was written. The zeal of thine house hath eaten me up" Zeal is defined as eagerness and ardent interest in pursuit of something and the passion for zeal means intense emotion compelling action and to put forth such effort. Now that have the understanding that my purpose on this earth is to do the will of my Father, my determination is to act on what I believe in His Word.

- Through His written and spoken word
- Through your thoughts
- Through your conversations
- Through your circumstances

I will praise the Lord for the rest of my days; nothing will stop I am determined to go all the way. While writing this book I began to get healed from things and became stronger because of the anointing and I prayed that everyone that rewards this book will be healed and delivered from anything that has them bound or sick. Jesus is our healer!

Never Under Estimate Yourself

Never underestimate yourself, it seem as though God is not big enough to carry you. The word (Under Estimate) cost underestimation is defined as the act of assessing the cost of a future venture lower than what actually cost. Cost underestimation causes cost overrun. Your life is very valuable to God. There are powers on the inside of every child of God. In every human soul on this earth there is a search of meaning, purpose significance and value. No matter what race, culture, language or religion this preoccupation with the need to find answer to their existence is in every human spirit.

What is Purpose

What is purpose? Purpose is reason for existence: the reason for which something exists or for which it has been done or made. Many people doubt this saying but I believe once you know who you are and the purpose of your life nothing can stop you. Hebrews 11:6 "But without faith it is impossible to please him: for he that cometh to God must believe that he is and that he is a rewarder of them that diligently seek him". Philippians 4:13" I can do all things through Christ which strengtheneth me". Christ's power and grace rest upon a believer to enable you to do all things that He ask of you to do. Our salvation comes as a gift of God's grace, but it can only be appropriate by the human response to faith. Saving faith in Jesus Christ is the only condition God requires for salvation. Faith is not only a profession about Christ, but also an activity coming from the heart of the child of who seek to follow Christ as Lord and Savior.

Passion

I was invited to minister at a conference in Florida at a church where the Word of God has so much impact. After I finished ministering there were some ladies that approaches me and told me how blesses their spirits were from the message. Getting home that afternoon I went ahead and took a nap. The glory of God rested upon me so heavily that I thought I was still in service. As I awakened it was a though Jesus was right in the room with me. As I went back to the church that I ministered at the pastors wife walked up to me and I began to thank her for inviting me and taking care of my expenses. One of my passions that I developed is to pray for people that I come in contact with, because you never know when you are going to need someone to pray for you.

What is Passion?

Passion is a gift of the spirit combined with the totality of all the experiences we've lived through. Passion is a gift of the spirit combined with the totality of all the experiences we've lived through. It endows each of us with the power to live and communicate with unbridled enthusiasm. Passion is most evident when the mind, body and spirit work together to create, develop and articulate or make manifest our feelings, ideas and most sacred values .Passion enables us to overcome obstacles (both real and imagined) and to see the world as a place of infinite potential.

Passion is the emotion of feeling very strongly about a subject or person.

Passion can also be used to refer to various forms of emotional suffering, and is often used in this context in Stoicism and some denominations of Buddhism

In Christianity, The Passion refers to the suffering of Jesus leading up to the Crucifixion.

It is good when others see things in you to confirm that God had been telling you all along. It amazes me because no one knows your heart but God.

Prayer

The message that I preached at the conference was titled "Ranks in Prayer" every child of God should pray, it is our duty to pray and to fast. The scriptures tell us in Luke 18:1 that we should pray and not faint. Jesus told His people to pray continually in order to accomplish God's will for their lives. If you lack in prayer God's will for your life will fade away. Looking back on life itself if I wasn't praying but others were praying for me I don't know where I would be. Nothing is impossible for God. Believe It or not life full of prayer makes life itself easier. Even when the devil puts stumbling block in your way, still pray.

References

1. Old and New Testament words meaning from the King James Bible

2. From Morris Cerullo God's Victorious Army Bible

3. Inserts from The Vines E. expository dictionary

4. Old and New Testament Thompson Chain Reference Study KJV Bible

5. The Full Life Study Bible

6. My own experience in life

2404341LV00001B/1/P
Printed in the USA
CPSIA information can be obtained at www.ICGtesting.com